The Greek Diet

Look and Feel Like a Greek God or Goddess
and Lose Up to Ten Pounds in Two Weeks

MARIA LOI
&
SARAH TOLAND

WILLIAM MORROW
An Imprint of HarperCollins*Publishers*

HarperCollins books may be purchased for educational, business, or sales promotional use. For information please e-mail the Special Markets Department at SPsales@harpercollins.com.

A hardcover edition of this book was published in 2015 by William Morrow, an imprint of HarperCollins Publishers.

FIRST WILLIAM MORROW PAPERBACK EDITION PUBLISHED 2016.

Designed by Lisa Stokes
Photographs © by Sasha Gitin

Library of Congress Cataloging-in-Publication Data has been applied for.

ISBN 978-0-06-233444-2

23 24 25 26 27 LBC 9 8 7 6 5

The Greek Diet

To the ancient Greeks, who recognized the beauty
in yogurt, olive oil, bread, and wine, and spread the
original Mediterranean diet to the rest of southern
Europe—and, eventually, the rest of the world

CONTENTS

INTRODUCTION

I T'S A WARM FRIDAY NIGHT in New York City, and people pack the sidewalks, winding briefcases and babies down walkways dotted by lindens and pin oaks. Taxis honk, trucks rattle through the side streets, and the clatter from open-air cafes spills out into the streets. Above the noise, brownstones and apartment buildings climb into the sky, while lines of skyscrapers sparkle with a million tiny lights. The city on a summer night is hot, noisy, and nearly maddening.

In one part of the city, though, there is something different, something almost calming and certainly nourishing—a sanctuary of sorts, a small Mediterranean oasis in the middle of the world's biggest and busiest city. This is the kitchen of Greek chef and restaurateur Maria Loi, known as the "Martha Stewart of Greece." This is where our story of the Greek Diet culminates, with plate after plate of delicious Mediterranean food that no one would guess was good for your body and waistline. But our story begins in a much different place, in ancient Greece, when history's most successful civilization founded democracy, philosophy, medicine, and, among these other things, the Mediterranean diet.

Most people who've been in a bookstore in the past ten years or recently flipped through a magazine know something of the Mediterranean diet. The unique plant-based nutritional approach has been ranked one of the healthiest diets in the world, proven to help lower cholesterol, thwart heart disease, and reduce the risk of nearly every chronic illness, including cancer, diabetes, and cognitive diseases like Alzheimer's. Few people know, though, that the healthiest diet in the world is also the easiest way to lose weight—easiest, that is, when you follow an authentic Mediterranean diet similar to the one created by the ancient Greeks.

Today, many versions of the Mediterranean diet abound, most of them distilled, hybridized, or distorted beyond what anyone, at any point in time, ate in any region of the Mediterranean basin. But fly to many areas of the Mediterranean today, and you'll find rates of obesity similar to those in the United States, where at least two-thirds of Americans are overweight or obese. Likewise, much of modern-day Greece, Italy, France, and Spain is now overweight, an unfortunate casualty of American cultural dominance. Many in the Mediterranean have exchanged their traditional way of eating for America's penchant for fast, processed, and otherwise fattening foods.

The book you've picked up is one of the few, if not only, on shelves today to leverage the real Mediterranean diet, based on the traditional Greek way of eating to help you lose weight. Science suggests the traditional Greek version of the Mediterranean diet is one of the healthiest and most slimming nutritional plans in the world. What makes our Greek Diet unique is that traditional Greek chef and ancient-dining expert Maria Loi shows you exactly how to follow the plan with authentic recipes that date back all the way to ancient Athens.

The Greek Diet combines Maria's intimate knowledge of the traditional Mediterranean diet with the expertise of longtime health journalist Sarah Toland to deliver a sustainable, easy-to-follow plan that can help anyone lose weight, no matter how much you've struggled in the past. *The Greek Diet* is one of the first books ever to use a traditional Greek Mediterranean diet to help people lose weight.

ABOUT THE AUTHORS

What do a world-renowned Greek chef and an American health journalist have in common? A lot, as it turns out, when it comes to how to eat to lose weight and boost health. That was the topic of conversation when we first met in Spring 2013. There, at a table crowded with plates of Maria's sumptuous food and surrounded by panoramic photographs of Greece, we discussed how most Americans had no idea that the foods we were eating at that moment—crusty bread with garlicky white beans, eggplant with cheese and nuts, grilled fish with olive-oiled wild greens, white and red wines—could be so rich and flavorful, yet so beneficial to your body and waistline. Sure, lots of Americans know that olive oil, red wine, and other staples of a traditional Mediterranean diet are good for overall health, but did they also know these mostly Greek foods could help burn fat better than low-carb shakes, energy bars, or frozen meals? At that point, the Greek Diet was born.

Maria Loi is one of the world's most celebrated Mediterranean chefs. Her renowned restaurant, Loi, in Manhattan attracted thousands of regular customers, from healthy eaters to burger lovers alike, along with celebrities, politicians, and some of New York's biggest power brokers. Maria's cooking has appeared on ABC's *Good Morning America,* the Food Network's *Restaurant Divided,* and *Not My Mama's Meal* with Bobby Deen. In 2012 she completed her own cooking series, *Cooking at Loi,* which aired on PBS stations nationwide. She has cooked at the White House for President Barack Obama, Vice President Joe Biden, and 250 guests. She currently serves as the ambassador of Greek food and Greek olive oil for the Chef's Club of Greece.

Maria was born in the small village of Thermo near the town of Nafpaktos, an area that was surrounded by mostly farmland at the time. Here, large families like Maria's passed culinary traditions down from generation to generation, sharing the secrets of how to make great Greek food—secrets that had survived since the days of the ancient Greeks. As a young woman, Maria left Thermo to pursue a career as a public affairs specialist and lobbyist. She quickly became a prominent lobbyist and businesswoman, traveling the world for large multinational companies like Texaco, Nokia, Sheraton Hotels, and Net Hold International.

After twenty years in big business, Maria was successful, but she wasn't happy. Her waistline had grown while her circle of friends had shrunk, and she didn't feel fulfilled, not in her own life nor with her nutrition. She retired from lobbying and returned to Nafpaktos, where she began cooking with family and friends. The experience was enlightening (and slimming) as she rediscovered that doing what she did as a little girl—learning, farming, and cooking—still made her immensely happy.

In 2002, she opened her first restaurant, Kouzina Maria Loi, in Nafpaktos. At the same time, she undertook an organized effort to learn as much as she could about the food of her ancestors and how her country's cuisine had originated. She studied and experimented, using her restaurant as a laboratory for new and exciting dishes based on older, healthier examples. In 2003, she was approached by a book committee for the 2004 Athens Olympic Games, who asked if she would write the official cookbook of the 2004 Summer Games, based on the ancient Mediterranean diet. She agreed, and today Maria's *Ancient Dining* remains one of the only authoritative sources on ancient Greek cuisine.

In 2011, Maria moved to New York City to open Loi in Manhattan, bringing the secrets of ancient Mediterranean cuisine across the ocean to share with a whole new audience of eager eaters. True to Maria's culinary ethics, whatever she makes is homemade from local, seasonal ingredients, and her food's balance of decadently rich and deliciously healthy ingredients has won her an international reputation.

Sarah Toland has worked as a health journalist for fifteen years, most recently as the senior health editor of *Men's Journal* magazine. She has appeared regularly as a health and fitness expert on Fox News Channel and other national networks and written on health for the *New York Times*, *Sports Illustrated*, *Delicious Living!*, *Trail Runner*, and *Mother Earth News*, among other publications. Prior to *Men's Journal*, Sarah was the senior editor of *Alternative Medicine* magazine, and the editor-in-chief of the national sports magazine *Inside Triathlon*.

Sarah's interest in health, nutrition, and fitness began as a young athlete in Cape Cod, Massachusetts, where she was born and raised. Surrounded by sand and sea, Sarah spent summers and winters outside, running along the beach, swimming in the ocean, and riding waves. By the time she graduated from college, Sarah was a five-time All-American in track and field and cross-country. She took her love of running to Boulder, Colorado, where she began training up to ninety miles a week and learned the hard way that proper nutrition was one of the only ways to excel. Within a year, Sarah was sponsored by Nike and had run Olympic qualifying times in the 5K and 10K. At the same time, she started a career as a journalist at Boulder's leading newspaper.

While Sarah went on to make several national teams, a trauma injury sidelined her running career shortly before the 2004 Olympic trials. She used her rehab time to swim and even worked a brief stint as a surf-rescue lifeguard in California. But her real love was journalism, and she continued to fuel her thirst for health and fitness by researching, reporting, and writing as much as she could on the subject for various publications. Today, Sarah continues to pursue her love of journalism in broadcast and print media while running up to sixty miles per week on a recreational basis.

THE GREEK DIET DEFINED

The Greek Diet uses a traditional Mediterranean style of eating to help readers lose weight easily and healthily, without starving, counting calories, or cutting out carbs, alcohol, fat, or other foods that make life worth living. The Greek Diet combines years of history, scientific study, and the recipes of authentic Mediterranean chef Maria Loi to create a diet that is truly Mediterranean.

The Greek Diet simplifies the complicated approach of most diet plans that use "points" or carb-counting and relies instead on twelve main "Pillar Foods"—twelve ingredients that research shows are imperative to fat-burning and disease prevention while increasing satiety and the overall culinary experience. We believe, as history shows, people not only have to enjoy the foods they eat to lose weight, but they also have to *savor* them in order to keep the weight off for good. For this reason, a component we call the "pleasure factor"— a food's ability to increase enjoyment and satisfaction—is a leading concept throughout this book.

Another fundamental component of the Greek Diet is preparing your own food. Many Westerners today don't cook, using the excuse of too little time or too high a cost. But studies show neither justification is an accurate perception: Cooking healthy food can take the same amount, if not less, time and money than it takes to run out to the drive-through. But the result of America's slow retreat from the kitchen has been a growing and deadly obesity epidemic, fueled by a relatively recent reliance on fast, packaged, or processed foods that are high in calories, sugar, and unhealthy fats, and low in nutrition.

Preparing and cooking your own meals is important to weight loss because it gives you direct control over what you eat, lessening the chances of your consuming toxic sugars, unhealthy fats, artificial additives, and other waist-widening chemicals. This book contains over 100 low-cost and authentic Mediterranean recipes designed to help you lose weight while enjoying delicious meals with friends and family. You don't have to cook every night, but the more you make your own food, the healthier and slimmer you'll be.

HOW TO USE THIS BOOK

Here's a liberating concept: You don't have to read *The Greek Diet* cover to cover to learn how to eat better to lose weight, prevent disease, boost energy, and overhaul your health. We encourage you to skim where you want to, and read deeply into the sections and chapters that interest you. Throughout this book, you'll also find helpful pull-out tips on how to use the twelve Pillar Foods to burn fat, increase flavor, and improve outward appearance.

This book is divided into four sections: Meet the Greeks, Going Greek, the Twelve Pillar Foods, and the Recipes. **Part I: Meet the Greeks** explains the history of the Mediterranean diet and why science has shown it to be a powerful antidote to stalled weight loss, low energy, and other health troubles.

Part II: Going Greek details how to start the Greek Diet while introducing you to the twelve Pillar Foods. This section includes a list of what to buy, what to toss, and what to keep in your pantry, along with meal plans and a one-week kick-start plan to lose up to five pounds in your first week on the diet. *If you choose to skim the book, we recommend reading this part more carefully to understand how to use the diet.*

Part III: The Twelve Pillar Foods explores the history, benefits, and culinary applications of each of the twelve Pillar Foods, explaining why these foods and drinks will help you lose weight. Each chapter in this section is divided into two distinct narratives:

- *The Sensual,* or Maria's experience growing up on an authentic Mediterranean diet and what we can learn about weight loss from the ancient Greeks; and
- *The Science,* written by Sarah, to show how the twelve Pillar Foods can suppress appetite, rev metabolism, stimulate fat burning, and help anyone lose the weight (and keep it off) for good.

Part IV: The Recipes feature over 100 easy-to-make meals, snacks, desserts, and drinks that use the twelve Pillar Foods to help you lose weight while enjoying mouthwatering homemade meals. While you don't have to try every (or any) recipe to lose weight, we recommend preparing your own meals and snacks from the Pillar Foods as often as possible. This will help speed your weight-loss efforts and, more importantly, turn the journey of losing weight into a life-changing discovery of the healthy and happy cook inside all of us.

PART I

MEET THE GREEKS

MEET THE GREEKS

SOMEWHERE OFF A TWISTING HIGHWAY, high in the mountains of central Greece, sit the ancient ruins of Delphi. The site, believed by the Greeks to be the center of Earth, is the size of a small village, spread out in temples, statues, and stone stadiums on the southern spur of Mount Parnassus. There is an amphitheater, a gymnasium, even a running track. From here, you can see the rugged mountains of the Pindos range, cut by fertile valleys of olive groves that once fed an entire civilization, and cupped by the Corinthian Gulf, still teeming with fish and birds.

But Delphi's main attraction in the days of the ancient Greeks wasn't its view, but a circular temple built in marble and limestone over a sacred spring. This is the oracle of Delphi, once the most sought-after shrine in the world. For centuries, hundreds of thousands of people from across the Mediterranean basin made pilgrimages to ask the oracle questions about their future and fate. Today, much of the oracle's sanctuary remains, with the same sweeping view of mountains and valleys that the curious and forsaken saw thousands of years ago.

Several thousand years later, the oracle of Delphi, as a symbol of all of ancient Greece, is still a source of answers about our future and fate. From ancient Greece we get nearly every facet of Western civilization that has made us successful, including our understanding of government, medicine, philosophy, art, and urban infrastructure. Today, doctors and researchers are just beginning to understand that the ancient Greeks also invented the world's most successful, health-giving, and slimming diet. This way of eating is called the Mediterranean diet.

Yet the true Mediterranean diet has unfortunately been distilled into a number of different versions by weight-loss books, nutrition gurus, and TV cooking shows. The diet has been so hybridized that it is no longer effective.

This is why we created the Greek Diet: to share the original principles of the Mediterranean diet that made the ancient Greeks so healthy and thin. But to understand the world's oldest and most effective diet, we first have to go back to the original source: ancient Greece.

MEET THE GREEKS

What kind of body do you want? Chances are, you wouldn't mind looking like one of those beautiful sculptures from ancient Greece. The men are lean and muscular; the women are slender and toned, with just the right delicate touch of feminine curve. Their bodies are undoubtedly breathtaking, and in today's Western world, where two-thirds of people are overweight or obese, these bodies are rare objets d'art, to be envied and ogled. Hundreds of these statues exist today, having survived the centuries from ancient Greece. Recently a popular museum exhibit, aptly named "The Body Beautiful in Ancient Greece," showed off the ancient Greek physique to millions internationally at the world's most eminent museums.

It's incredible that the ancient Greeks were able to capture physical human perfection in stone, marble, and bronze. But art historians have long recognized that there was no possible way the ancient Greeks achieved the fine detail exhibited by their sculptures from imagination alone. While some artists certainly idealized and added aesthetic impressions to enhance their work, the ancient Greeks largely modeled statues on people living at the time.

The truth is, body fat was hard to find in ancient Greece. Researchers know this not only from surviving artwork, but also from thousands of other artifacts the highly successful culture left behind. We know from their ancient written records that the Greeks valued athletics and physical upkeep; the philosopher Aristotle wrote that the most beautiful bodies in the world were those "capable of enduring all efforts, either of the racecourse or of bodily strength." We know the ancient Greeks invented the Olympic Games and the world's first gymnasium, along with a number of modern-day sports like wrestling and marathon running. They were the first society in history to identify obesity as a medical disease and to shun it, associating the condition of being overweight with the socioeconomic curse of being low-class.

Yet despite that many in ancient Greece were lean—far leaner than in today's Greece or the rest of the Western world—they didn't deny themselves their pleasures, cut out food groups, or spend great lengths of time at the gymnasium or on sports. On the contrary, this is the same culture that invented the concept of public leisure baths and the symposium, a giant party for drinking, eating, and discussing ideas. The ancient Greeks drank wine copiously and are credited with introducing the wine habit to the rest of Europe. Perhaps most strikingly, the Greeks ate an extremely high-fat diet—higher in fat than what the average overweight American eats today. The Greeks also indulged in bread and other grains, and consumed full-fat dairy, alongside honey and nuts. In short, the ancient Greeks liked to eat and did so often, enjoying nearly every "forbidden food" of dieters today—carbs, fat, dairy, gluten, sugar, and alcohol—while staying wonderfully thin.

The ancient Greeks were lean without trying to be so, and what is even more surprising is that the ancient Greeks managed to stay thin even though they lived in a world similar to that of most Westerners with weight problems today. The ancient Greeks also had access to many of the modern-day foods we do, including grains, dairy, sugar, and other perceived culprits of the obesity epidemic. Even more notable, the ancient Greeks consumed these foods on a regular basis, with great enjoyment and an insatiable appetite that would shock most yo-yo dieters and weight-loss junkies today.

THE ANCIENT GREEK DIET

The ancient Greeks' diet can be summarized in four words: bread, wine, olive oil, and plants. While wealthier Greeks could afford to enjoy a variety of cuisines, these four foods were the mainstays of their meals. For breakfast, lunch, and dinner, they ate fresh bread baked from wheat or barley, often dipped in wine. This staple was served with fruit, vegetables, or beans, the latter two seasoned with herbs, spices, and, of course, olive oil. The Greeks also ate nuts and plenty of seafood from the blue-silk waters of the Mediterranean Sea; their drink of choice was wine, often consumed at all three meals, even breakfast, but diluted with water to be made less potent. The ancients raised poultry, including pheasant and quail, but they valued the birds more for their eggs than their meat. Red meat was a rarity, and when it was consumed, the Greeks ate lean game meat, like boar, rabbit, and goat. Unlike latter-day Europeans, the ancients didn't typically use butter and milk in cooking, but they did enjoy cheese, honey, figs, and fermented milk products similar to modern-day Greek yogurt. However, the Greeks followed a very temperate diet, eating most foods according to Maria's favorite native adage, *metron ariston*: "Everything in moderation."

There was perhaps one exception to the *metron ariston* rule: olive oil. The ancient Greeks consumed a tremendous amount of olive oil—a habit that continued through history until only several decades ago, when the people of Greece began eating a more Americanized diet of imported fast and packaged goods. But before then, the people of Greece had a high intake of olive oil, more than any other people around the world, including anywhere in the Mediterranean. For example, when the famous Seven Countries Study was completed in the 1970s—one of the first large-scale research efforts to examine the effects of diet on health—it was found that the mid-twentieth-century Cretans were getting an impressive one-third of their daily calories from the oil. But as we'll soon see, olive oil, high in healthy fat, is the secret to burning body fat, filling you up and increasing your body's metabolism and ability to oxidize fat, all while helping to prevent heart disease and boost overall health.

THE GREEK DIET TODAY

Fast forward a few thousand years: What the ancient Greeks ate is now called the Mediterranean diet, per the Seven Countries Studies and based on what the people of Crete ate in the 1950s and '60s. We call this diet the Greek Diet, based on Maria Loi's Greek heritage and culinary success, and to differentiate our plan from ineffective and hybridized versions of the modern Mediterranean diet.

The Greek Diet is made up of many of the same staples the ancient Greeks enjoyed: fresh vegetables, fruits, beans, whole grains, herbs, nuts, wine, and seafood. What makes this diet unique—and very Greek? The primary macronutrient in the Greek Diet is fat, with up to forty percent of daily calories coming from the heart-healthy monounsaturated fats and other lipids found in olive oil. We'll discuss the benefits of the healthy fats in olive oil in greater length in Pillar One, but briefly, monounsaturated fat (MUFA) has been shown to increase our fat oxidization, or the body's ability to use fat as a fuel source. What's more, a certain type of MUFA called oleic acid has been shown to curb hunger while increasing feelings of fullness, or satiety. Olive oil also has a number of specific properties that speed weight loss.

The Greek Diet is also high in protein, but not the kind of protein that many Westerners eat: industrially raised red meat rich in waist-thickening saturated fats; processed chicken that's fried or prepared in high-sugar, high-carbohydrate sauces; or lastly, the synthetic proteins found in energy bars, smoothies, and shakes. Instead, the Greek Diet is rich in lean protein from seafood, beans, nuts, and yogurt, each of which has specific benefits shown to help us lose weight. Unlike common American diet protein sources, every type of protein we eat on the Greek Diet includes a powerful advantage to your waistline:

- Yogurt contains healthy bacteria known as probiotics shown to fuel metabolism and accelerate fat burning.
- Seafood contains marine omega-3 fatty acids shown to accelerate fat-burning and prevent disease.
- Beans contain *natural* soluble and insoluble fiber shown to increase satiety and balance blood sugar.
- Nuts contain a variety of micronutrients shown to lower blood sugar while increasing metabolism and satiety.

The Greek Diet contains little to no red meat, which large-scale population studies have shown can cause a normal person to gain one pound per year without any other changes to diet.

YES, YOU CAN EAT CARBS

Just as important to the Greek Diet as protein are complex carbohydrates found in plants, including vegetables, fruits, nuts, and whole grains. Every major population study, including the China-Cornell-Oxford Project detailed in the renowned *The China Study,* has found that a primarily plant-based diet high in micronutrient-rich plant foods helps prevent nearly every significant disease and ailment, including weight gain and obesity. Additionally, the complex carbs found in plant foods, specifically whole grains, provide a critical source of energy imperative for a healthy metabolism while helping us feel full and, more important, happy.

If you're thinking that there's no way you can lose weight eating bread and pasta, you're right: You can't lose weight eating the refined, processed breads and pasta typical of the Standard American Diet (with the appropriate acronym SAD). Instead, you lose weight eating the type of healthy *whole-grain* bread, pasta, and cereals that have been enjoyed by those in Greece and all over the Mediterranean for centuries, since the days of the ancient Greeks. These unprocessed whole grains, including 100 percent whole wheat bread, oatmeal, whole-grain pasta, and quinoa, are higher in fiber and lower in sugar than refined grains like enriched white bread, enriched pasta, crackers, and sugary breakfast cereals. Additionally, on the Greek Diet, we eat whole grains the way the ancient Greeks did: Not with sugary processed tomato sauce or unhealthy fats like butter or hydrogenated vegetable oils, but with lots of metabolism-boosting olive oil, which also helps balance the body's hormonal response to the sugars found in food.

YES, YOU CAN DRINK ALCOHOL (WINE, THAT IS)

On the Greek Diet, it's not just about what you eat, but what you drink, too. The ancient Greeks were renowned for their enjoyment of wine. Today, studies show the Greeks' favorite drink not only helps protect the heart, but it also helps speed weight-loss efforts by amazingly increasing the body's caloric burn while lowering blood-sugar levels to thwart the fat-storing hormone insulin. Similarly, coffee, and tea, consumed daily by the ancient Greeks, also play an important role in weight loss by significantly speeding metabolism, increasing satiety, and balancing blood-sugar levels.

EMPHASIZING THE PLEASURE FACTOR OF FOOD

As is true of any nutritional plan, what the Greek Diet does *not* include is as significant as the foods it does. Nowhere in ancient Greece or anywhere else in the Mediterranean (until a few decades ago, when Greeks, Italians, French, and other Mediterranean peoples began importing Americanized eating habits) were there processed and refined foods like packaged breads, rolls, chips, cookies, crackers, frozen diet dinners, energy bars, and sugar-sweetened yogurt. You won't find these foods—along with soda, energy drinks, or sugary coffee drinks—anywhere in the Greek Diet. Almost all processed foods and drinks contain sugar, unhealthy fats, and/or artificial and chemical preservatives, flavorings, and colors that have been linked to hormone imbalance, weight gain, and obesity. We believe simply cutting out packaged and processed foods can cause most people to lose five to ten pounds, without changing anything else about their diets!

The Greek Diet accomplishes all this while emphasizing what we call the pleasure factor—how much we enjoy foods. No weight-loss diet should force you to give up the tastes, textures, and effects of nourishing foods and drinks that we believe make life worth living. On the Greek Diet, we encourage you to eat a large amount of healthy fat, along with creamy yogurt, fresh vegetables, sweet whole fruit, crunchy nuts, and filling breads, pasta, and other whole-grain foods. We want you to enjoy a cup of coffee with breakfast and a glass of wine with dinner, and we want you to eat dessert. You don't have to cut out carbs, gluten, or any other food group to lose weight, and you don't have to count calories or restrict your intake. As research has shown, the key to significant and long-term weight loss is feeling happy, healthy, and good about yourself and about what you eat—not hungry, miserable, and deprived.

The Science Behind the Greek Diet

One of the most important studies ever conducted on how to lose weight—a study that changed the national conversation on the best way to burn fat—surprised many low-carb fanatics when it concluded a true Mediterranean diet was the best way to drop fat while improving overall health. The study, conducted by Israeli scientists and published in the eminent *New England Journal of Medicine* in 2008, was one of the first large-scale research projects to compare the three most popular diets of the past three decades: (1) the low-carb or Atkins diet, which peaked in popularity in the early part of the 2000s; (2) the low-fat diet, recommended by the U.S. government and American Heart Association since the 1980s; and (3) a traditional Mediterranean diet, defined by the Seven Countries Study.

After two years of extensive research on more than 300 people, the study's results were impressive: Those on a true Mediterranean diet lost far more weight than those on a low-fat diet, and they were healthier than those who had eaten the Atkins diet. The study also found that participants on a true Mediterranean diet had a much easier time sticking with the diet—and, thereby, actually losing weight—than those who followed the low-carb approach, many of whom had to drop off the diet before the study's end.

The effect was so dramatic, in fact, that a doctor who analyzed the study's results told the media, "If any primary care physician . . . has a patient on the Atkins diet two years on, you should probably find that patient and . . . find out how they did it. I've not seen anyone in my practice who is still on the diet two years later. Compliance past a few months is the number one problem with the Atkins diet." The same doctor added, "The Mediterranean diet is the one I find patients are most likely to maintain long-term compliance with."

There are also countless other studies showing a wide range of health benefits to adopting the traditional Mediterranean diet, including a reduction in the risk of many common chronic diseases like cancer, diabetes, Alzheimer's, Parkinson's, arthritis, and the number one killer, heart disease. Research also shows the Mediterranean diet can help lower LDL ("bad") cholesterol, even more so than taking prescription statin drugs. The diet also has an overwhelming number of cognitive benefits, including improving overall brain health, increasing focus, and fighting depression. Finally, the diet has been shown to increase fertility, improve breathing function, boost eye health, lower the risk of birth defects, and reduce the number of dental problems. For these reasons, a traditional *Greek* Mediterranean diet is the preferred nutritional approach by many of the world's top medical institutions, including Harvard Medical School and Oldways, the premier nutritional think tank in the United States.

PART II

GOING GREEK

GOING GREEK

IN THIS SECTION, we share with you how to "go Greek": how to implement the easy and enjoyable Greek Diet today so you can start down the incredible life-changing path to lasting, sustainable weight loss and better overall health. In this section you'll learn:

- The twelve Pillar Foods that will help you fight fat and chronic disease
- How to start the diet
- Which foods to stock up on and which foods to throw out
- What to eat the first week for breakfast, lunch, and dinner
- How much you can eat
- How much weight you can expect to lose
- How to kick-start your weight loss—a plan to lose up to five pounds in one week
- Cooking—and not cooking—on the Greek Diet
- Staying Greek on the go
- Gluten- and dairy-free alternatives
- Exercise
- Other weight-loss aids
- What to do if you don't see results
- Meal plans

Eating and losing weight on the Greek Diet is a simple two-step process:

1. Stop eating processed and refined foods and drinks.

2. Start eating the most delicious, health-giving foods on the planet: the twelve Pillar Foods.

WHAT ARE THE TWELVE PILLAR FOODS?

In classical Greek mythology, there were twelve great gods, known as the Olympians, who ruled the Greek pantheon from Mount Olympus, changing history and the fate of the Greek people forever.

Similarly, on the Greek Diet, there are twelve Pillar Foods that can dramatically change your body, mood, and health:

- Olive oil
- Yogurt
- Vegetables
- Beans
- Seafood
- Whole grains
- Wine
- Herbs and spices
- Fruit
- Coffee and tea
- Nuts and seeds
- Chicken and eggs

The Pillar Foods appear in approximate order of importance, but what matters more than how often you eat them is that you do *eat* them, enjoying most Pillar Foods on a daily basis, including olive oil, yogurt, vegetables, beans, whole grains, wine, herbs and spices, and coffee and tea.

GETTING STARTED

Trying to adopt a new way of eating is always difficult, no matter how delicious or life-changing a different diet may be. Everyone has certain dietary habits and patterns, preferring food that may not necessarily taste better or make us feel good for the simple reason we've become so accustomed to it and the routines surrounding that food. Research shows most dieters who try to adopt a totally new way of eating in one day—and expect to stick with it—fail miserably after just a few days. If you currently eat mostly packaged, processed, and/or fast foods, or if very few Pillar Foods are part of your nutritional repertoire now, you may want to start the Greek Diet with small steps, changing one or two things about what you eat and drink every day for at least a week. For example, the first day or two, stop drinking soda and switch your daily energy drink to a cup of coffee instead. Several days later, replace crackers, potato chips, and other snack foods in your diet with a cup of Greek yogurt, a piece of fruit, a handful of nuts, and/or vegetables dipped in hummus. When you have removed most of the processed foods from your diet—and added more of the Pillar Foods—you'll be ready to adopt the diet in its entirety.

If you already eat somewhat healthfully and/or your current diet includes a handful of the Pillar Foods, you're ready to go full speed ahead on the Greek Diet. Choose a day to begin the diet, preferably during a day you work if you're employed: Pairing a new eating plan with a structured work schedule can make it easier to adopt a new routine. The day before, stock your refrigerator and pantry with the following foods if you don't already have them. Include enough for approximately one week of meals.

THE GREEK DIET SHOPPING LIST

- High-quality extra-virgin olive oil (the investment is worth it!)
- Greek yogurt, preferably plain with 2% fat
- Any fresh and frozen vegetables (broccoli, spinach, kale, cauliflower, tomatoes, eggplant, carrots, lettuce, sweet potatoes)
- Canned and/or dried beans (chickpeas, lentils, white beans, black beans, kidney beans)
- Any fresh whole fruit (apples, pears, strawberries, raspberries, bananas, grapes, oranges, grapefruit, peaches, plums)
- Dried herbs and spices (oregano, thyme, basil, cumin, rosemary, cayenne, ginger, cinnamon, nutmeg, sea salt)
- Three servings of fresh or frozen seafood (salmon, cod, tilapia, canned tuna, shrimp, scallops)
- Lemons (to flavor plain water and for preparing salads and seafood)
- High-quality balsamic vinegar (for salads and cooking)
- Onions, shallots, or leeks (imperative for cooking anything!)
- Whole grains for cooking (oatmeal, wheat berries, barley, quinoa, farro, brown rice)

- Whole-grain pasta (see page 112 to learn how to be sure you're getting whole grains)
- Whole-grain bread (100 percent whole wheat, whole oat, whole rye, whole pumpernickel; see page 112)
- Roasted or raw nuts (almonds, cashews, peanuts, walnuts, pecans)
- 100 percent nut butters, without added sugar
- Whole-grain flour (whole wheat, spelt, cornmeal, oat; see page 111)
- Eggs
- One or two servings of chicken, preferably organic
- Coffee, preferably caffeinated
- Black or herbal tea
- Wine (red or white)
- Honey
- Organic milk (for coffee, tea, and yogurt making)
- Feta and ricotta cheeses (for cooking)

As you stock your kitchen, should you get rid of food that's not part of the Greek Diet? Ideally, your cabinets and fridge will be big enough to store both, helping to lessen the impression that you're drastically changing your eating habits while offering a safety net to sneak a potato chip or cookie as you adapt to a new diet (recognizing we're human, after all, helps reduce the physiological and psychological hold that many temptation foods can have over us). Eventually, you'll be ready to clear these foods out of your cabinet, whether it takes you a week, a month, or several months. However, some of us are ready for a drastic change or may feel tempted by the mere presence of certain foods not on the Greek Diet plan if they remain in the kitchen. If either case describes you, donate the following to your local food pantry:

- Generic vegetable oils, margarine, and butter
- Packaged snacks (pretzels, potato chips, cookies, crackers, fruit leathers, energy bars, granola bars)
- Packaged breads, rolls, tortillas, and other bread products that aren't 100 percent whole grain
- Sugar-sweetened yogurt
- Processed cheese (American)

- Breakfast cereals (with the exception of whole-grain cereals, see page 112 to learn how to be sure you're getting whole grains)
- Red meat
- Frozen snacks (waffles, pizzas, tater tots, ice cream)
- Frozen dinners
- Ketchup, bottled salad dressings, sugary barbecue and tomato sauces
- White flours
- White sugar, brown sugar, agave, and other refined sweeteners
- Soda, juice, and other high-sugar-content beverages

THE FIRST WEEK

Congratulations. You've stocked your pantry with fresh, delicious, slimming foods that will overhaul your mood and boost your health. And maybe you've also cleared out all the unhealthy stuff that can sabotage your waistline. Now, you're ready to start Day One on the Greek Diet. But how do you begin? The answer is easy: Start eating more Pillar Foods. When do you begin? With breakfast on the very first day you decide to start on your new weight-loss adventure.

Breakfast

Start your day with a glass of water to rehydrate the body, with a splash of lemon to help detoxify your system. Then it's time to prepare breakfast. Don't make the mistake of thinking you can save calories by not eating a morning meal. Research shows breaking the overnight fast helps jump-start your metabolism and balances hunger hormones that, left unchecked, can sabotage your best weight-loss intentions by four in the afternoon. Studies have also found that those who eat a healthy breakfast that includes some protein lose more weight more quickly than those who don't. One of the healthiest foods highest in hunger-stopping protein that you can eat for breakfast is Greek yogurt. As we'll detail in Pillar Two: Yogurt, this rich and creamy treat is higher in protein than regular yogurt, even eggs—one cup of Greek yogurt has more than 3 times the protein of a single egg! Pair a cup of cold yogurt with a tablespoon of nuts, a bit of whole-grain muesli, and/or fresh fruit. Or for a savory, satiating meal, try a cup of yogurt with a half teaspoon of olive oil and fresh herbs.

If you don't like yogurt, don't worry: You can still follow the Greek Diet. There are many other high-protein breakfast foods, including eggs, oatmeal (1 cup of instant or rolled oats has 6 grams of protein, the same as in an egg), or Maria's favorite, a Greek frittata, or omelet, made with vegetables and herbs (and, preferably, Greek yogurt too!). For more options, see our meal plans on page 29.

Another part of your morning meal, whether you drink it before, during, or after breakfast, should be a cup of hot coffee or tea, preferably caffeinated. We like to drink coffee or tea while making breakfast! The antioxidants and caffeine in either help kick-start the body's metabolism while warming and energizing you for the day. The healthiest way to take your cup of coffee or tea is with a splash of organic milk to help balance the acid in coffee and tea. But avoid adding sugar, which boosts blood sugar levels, and artificial sweeteners, which contain toxins that can stimulate appetite and interfere with the body's hormone levels.

Lunch and Dinner

On the Greek Diet, the more plants you eat, the healthier and slimmer you'll be. Plant foods, especially low-calorie, high-fiber vegetables, should be the main focus of your afternoon and evening meals, with at least 50 percent of your plate dedicated to nonstarchy options like kale, spinach, salad greens, broccoli, cauliflower, eggplant, carrots, cabbage, artichokes, Brussels sprouts, peppers, and celery—the options are limitless. This doesn't mean, though, that you should eat salads for lunch and dinner every day. When you learn to make your own meals with Maria according to a true Mediterranean diet, there are a variety of delicious vegetable-based dishes to enjoy, including lasagna, moussaka, stews, pies, casseroles, and more.

Whether you eat a salad or spinach quiche for lunch, or enjoy vegetables with shrimp or chicken and rice for dinner, use olive oil to dress or cook the dishes you make or prepare. This ensures that you eat a generous daily amount of the fat-burning oil, helping curb hunger, balance blood sugar, and increase the body's metabolic burn.

In most Western diets, animal meat is the main entrée of every lunch and dinner. But as research shows, this habit has helped Westerners pack on the pounds; studies have concluded that people who eat large amounts of fatty animal meat weigh more and gain more weight than those who don't. One large British study of close to 400,000 people found that for every 450 calories of meat that research participants ate daily, they gained 4 pounds over a 5-year period!

For this reason, it's important to rethink what role animal protein plays on your plate, shifting your focus from red meat and pork to proteins proven to slim your waistline: low-fat dairy (Greek yogurt), beans, seafood, eggs, and chicken. Add beans and yogurt liberally to your daily meals, eat seafood and eggs three to four times each per week, and use chicken in your meals approximately twice a week.

The rest of your lunch and dinner plates should include a healthy whole grain, whether that's brown rice, whole wheat pasta, whole-grain bread (the ancient Greeks' favorite!), farro, quinoa, barley, or another cooked cereal grain. Whole grains not only give your body the complex carbs it needs for energy and proper hormone and metabolic function, they also provide a significant amount of protein. Quinoa boasts 4 grams of filling protein per ½ cup, while the same serving of whole-grain pasta contains approximately 5 grams.

Snacks

Not all diets encourage snacking, but we believe keeping your stomach full and happy with a small snack between meals is integral to consistent, long-term weight loss. That said, how we snack on the Greek Diet is radically different from how most Westerners snack: tearing into a sugary granola or energy bar; reaching mindlessly into a bag of chips, pretzels, or cookies; or opting for some other refined high-sugar, high-carb snack, like a bowl of sugary cereal or piece of refined-flour pizza.

We encourage snacking on the Greek Diet the same way traditional Greeks snacked—a piece of fruit here, a handful of nuts there, or perhaps a small cup of creamy, filling Greek yogurt. Having a *small* snack once or twice between meals during the day can help stoke your metabolism and prevent overeating, especially at night when most dieters can succumb to dangerous bingeing.

Also, there is nothing wrong with a cup of coffee or tea for a snack during the day or after dinner. Caffeinated coffee and tea throughout the day can help boost your metabolism and fuel an afternoon workout; a cup of decaffeinated coffee or tea after dinner helps increase feelings of satiety and satisfaction.

Water

Drink up to eight 8-ounce glasses of water daily to stay hydrated and keep your metabolism firing. Water is also important to keep you feeling full: Many people mistake thirst for hunger and end up overeating for no reason other than they forgot to drink water! Plain water with a slice of lemon or lime is best, but carbonated water with a splash of fresh grapefruit, orange, or cranberry juice will do if you're craving a sweet drink. Whatever you do, avoid soda (both diet and regular) and juice, which add empty calories and send your blood sugar through the roof.

Wine

A glass or two of wine with dinner provides important antioxidants that help boost metabolism and the body's fat-burning abilities, and protect your heart. Wine also plays into what we call the *pleasure factor,* helping increase the flavor of food as well as your overall enjoyment of meals and social dinners while you lose weight. While it's not necessary that you drink wine on the Greek Diet, if you already enjoy wine, continuing to do so will only speed your weight-loss efforts. Just remember that more than two glasses of wine daily can have the opposite effect, causing weight gain. For more on how wine aids in weight loss, see Pillar Seven: Wine.

Dessert

Dessert is not off-limits on the Greek Diet. Quite the opposite, we encourage you to have an after-dinner snack. We believe, as research shows, that knowing you can have a small snack after dinner prevents overeating during dinner, as well as late-night binge-eating after dinner, a common and disastrous habit among many dieters.

What's more, we designed the Greek Diet so that you can follow it for life, not just for a few weeks or months. And who wants to give up sweet treats indefinitely? Well, you don't have to in order to lose weight: Desserts have been enjoyed by healthy populations, including the ancient Greeks, for centuries, and research shows enjoying a small treat daily can help you stay the course of any weight-loss plan for longer periods of time. There's only one caveat: You have to make your own dessert out of the Pillar Foods, whether that's healthy whole-grain flours, nuts, fruit, or, our favorite, delicious Greek yogurt. And be sure to keep your serving sizes reasonable, not the supersized pieces of cake, cookies, and other sweets you see at restaurants, bakeries, and in grocery stores. For dessert suggestions with serving sizes, see our meal plans on page 38.

HOW MUCH CAN I EAT?

In most diet plans, this is the big question, as dieters immediately want to know how much they're allowed in order to still lose weight. On the Greek Diet, we provide guidelines with exact measurements for each meal in our meal plans on pages 38–46. At first glance, it may seem difficult to adhere to these sizes, but trust us: You won't want more. The Pillar Foods are so satiating and pleasurable, especially if cooked according to Maria's recipes, you'll be too full to eat more.

Still, we are used to overeating: In most modern Western countries, plate and portion sizes are too big, and we've grown accustomed to eating gigantic muffins, oversized salads, supersized sandwiches, big-plated dinners, and dessert, on top of a continual cycle of snack foods and jumbo drinks throughout the day. It's important to break the cycle of mindless eating if you want to lose weight. The best way to do this is to find out why you're continuing to eat past your hunger point: Are you bored? Do you feel lonely, angry, or stressed by the day? Are you unhappy? Do you crave social interaction that long meals provide? Are you distracted by the TV, computer, or your work? When you find your trigger for overeating—and you can have different triggers at different meals or times of the day—develop an alternative other than food that can calm the trigger. For example, if you overeat because you feel lonely, call a friend instead of continuing to pile your plate with food. If you eat too much snack food at work because you're stressed, use the 10 minutes you'd normally take to go to the vending machine and cram down some chips to take a short walk around the block, breathing in deeply through your nose and out through your mouth.

Ultimately, we believe the key to long-lasting weight loss is learning to eat meals only when you're hungry (as long as you eat three meals per day, avoiding the bad habit of bingeing when hungry) and to stop eating *before* you're full. Although they're not Greek, the Okinawans of traditional Japan, most of whom are very thin, have an old saying, *hara hachi bu*, "Eat only until you're 80 percent full." Eating until you're stuffed means you've consumed too much, as it takes your brain several minutes to realize you're full. The habit also stretches your stomach, making you want more food the next time you eat, causing a vicious cycle of overeating that will sabotage any diet plan.

HOW MUCH WEIGHT WILL I LOSE?

If your current diet comprises a lot of fast food and/or processed, refined, packaged junk, you'll most likely drop several pounds in the first week simply by swapping Pillar Foods for these items. After that, you can expect to lose at least one to two pounds per week, which is ideal for sustainable weight loss. If you find you're losing more than two pounds per week, increase your intake of the Pillar Foods to prevent slowing your body's metabolism and causing other detrimental effects inherent in overly rapid weight loss, including the strong potential for rapid weight *gain*.

KICK-START YOUR WEIGHT LOSS WITH THE TWO-WEEK YOGURT PLAN

If you're anxious for results and want to jump-start your weight loss by following a stricter plan for the first week, the following 1,200-calorie meal plan is designed to help you lose as much weight as is safely possible in two weeks. The plan does this by encouraging you to eat a bowl of satiating Greek yogurt instead of a full-course dinner every night. You will repeat the first week's menu for the second week; this helps make the plan easier to follow. For the plan to be effective, though, you should eat all snacks and meals, and drink a full glass of water with each meal and snack, or, alternatively, between every meal and snack. Like you'd do for any weight-loss plan, consult with your doctor before starting.

KICK-START YOGURT PLAN
Two-Week Kick-Start Meal Plan

Asterisk indicates recipe included.

	"Kick-Start" Breakfast	Mid-Morning Snack	Lunch	Afternoon Snack	Dinner
SUNDAY	Greek Frittata* OR Any omelet made with 2 eggs and vegetables of different colors AND Coffee or tea	1 cup raspberries AND Greek mountain tea	Baked Salmon with Yogurt Sauce* AND Marouli Salad with Feta-Yogurt Dressing*	1 orange	Eat 1 cup 2% plain Greek yogurt, and drink 1 cup mountain tea and water every night this week for dinner

TOTAL: 1,200 calories, 72 grams protein

	"Kick-Start" Breakfast	Mid-Morning Snack	Lunch	Afternoon Snack	Dinner
MONDAY	1 bowl oatmeal made with ¼ cup dry steel cut oats and water, topped with ½ cup fresh sliced peaches and ¼ cup chopped walnuts AND Coffee or tea	1 cup cantaloupe cubes AND Greek mountain tea	Couscous Salad* AND Grilled Chicken Breast*	1 cup blackberries	Eat 1 cup 2% plain Greek yogurt, and drink 1 cup mountain tea and water every night this week for dinner

TOTAL: 1,200 calories, 85 grams protein

	"Kick-Start" Breakfast	Mid-Morning Snack	Lunch	Afternoon Snack	Dinner
TUESDAY	Scrambled Eggs with Feta Cheese (Kayana)* AND 1 medium orange AND Coffee or tea	½ cup 2% plain Greek yogurt topped with ½ cup blueberries and ½ oz. walnuts (7 halves) AND Greek mountain tea	Lentil Salad with Oranges* OR Any salad made with leafy greens and beans, lentils, or nuts	1 cup cherries	Eat 1 cup 2% plain Greek yogurt, and drink 1 cup mountain tea and water every night this week for dinner

TOTAL: 1,200 calories, 72 grams protein

	"Kick-Start" Breakfast	Mid-Morning Snack	Lunch	Afternoon Snack	Dinner
WEDNESDAY	¾ cup 2% plain Greek yogurt topped with 1 oz. (14 halves)chopped walnuts, ½ cup sliced strawberries and ½ cup blackberries AND Coffee or tea	1 medium apple AND Greek mountain tea	Lentil Soup (Fakes)*	1 oz. (about 1 handful) almonds	Eat 1 cup 2% plain Greek yogurt, and drink 1 cup mountain tea and water every night this week for dinner

TOTAL: 1,200 calories, 77 grams protein

	"Kick-Start" Breakfast	Mid-Morning Snack	Lunch	Afternoon Snack	Dinner
THURSDAY	Greek Morning Shake (includes coffee)* AND 1 cup raspberries	1 medium peach AND Greek mountain tea	Greek Salad (Horiatiki Salata) with Cucumber Dressing* AND Grilled Chicken Breast* OR Takeout Greek salad with grilled chicken breast	1 cup blueberries	Eat 1 cup 2% plain Greek yogurt, and drink 1 cup mountain tea and water every night this week for dinner

TOTAL: 1,200 calories, 80 grams protein

FRIDAY	1 bowl oatmeal made with ¼ cup dry steel cut oats and water, topped with ½ cup fresh blackberries and ¼ cup slivered almonds AND Coffee or tea	1 oz. (about 1 handful or 14 halves) walnuts AND Greek mountain tea	Artichokes with Rice and Vegetables*	1 medium pear	Eat 1 cup 2% plain Greek yogurt, and drink 1 cup mountain tea and water every night this week for dinner

TOTAL: 1,200 calories, 58 grams protein

SATURDAY	Scrambled Eggs with Feta Cheese (Kayana)* AND ½ avocado AND Coffee or tea	¾ cup 2% plain Greek yogurt with ½ cup blackberries AND Greek mountain tea	Watermelon Salad with Feta and Mint* AND Stuffed Baby Eggplant (Papoutsakia)*	1 oz. pistachios	Eat 1 cup 2% plain Greek yogurt, and drink 1 cup mountain tea and water every night this week for dinner

TOTAL: 1,200 calories, 66 grams protein

Repeat the first week's menu for the second week.

DO I HAVE TO COOK?

Flip through this book and you'll discover dozens of beautiful recipes for delicious Greek and Mediterranean dishes made from our twelve health-giving, fat-busting Pillar Foods. We created these recipes with care to appeal to both working professionals and busy parents looking to feed their entire families; to those who haven't ever tasted a Greek dish before and those who adore Mediterranean cuisine; to those who aspire to be amateur chefs and those who barely know how to boil pasta. Many of the recipes are simple, made from relatively inexpensive ingredients you can easily get at any supermarket, and don't take longer to make than it takes to drive to a fast-food chain or takeout restaurant to pick up dinner.

Homemade meals and dishes on the Greek Diet aren't your typical diet recipes, either. There are no boring, tasteless low-fat recipes—baked chicken with broiled broccoli and rice, the bran muffins with applesauce instead of oil—that studies show don't help people lose weight. Nor are there any of the Atkins variety, with steak or chicken thighs only, or breakfasts made from just bacon and eggs—meals that aren't balanced, necessarily easy, or inexpensive to make, or reasonable to serve to friends and family. Finally, the recipes in this book call for almost no packaged ingredients: no popular processed diet products like margarine, low-calorie salad dressing, fat-free sour cream, artificial sugars—you get the point. They are simply healthy, balanced recipes made from natural health-giving whole foods and fats people have enjoyed for centuries—and that the majority of wide-scale research ever conducted on nutrition shows will help the average person lose weight.

But why cook in the first place? The answer to that question is manifold. First, studies show eating just one takeout or restaurant meal a week increases your chances of weight gain. That's because nearly all takeout food, frozen dinners, fast-food items, and even many sit-down restaurant meals are made with a high amount of unhealthy fats, refined grains, preservatives, and hidden sugar (many fast-food chains even add sugar to hamburgers and hamburger rolls!).

When you cook at home, even if you don't necessarily cook healthfully, chances are you're not using hydrogenated oils, preservatives, artificial flavorings, hidden sugars, and other detrimental ingredients that wreak havoc on your body. Instead, you have control over exactly what you and your family eat. And when you learn how easy and tasty it is to cook healthfully at home, a whole new world opens up: Food tastes better and you will begin to lose weight without even trying, simply because you've cut out all the unhealthy ingredients found in takeout and processed food that rack up your body's caloric intake and total toxic load.

Now, we know what you're thinking: You have no time to cook. We get it. You're busy with your job, kids, commuting, cleaning, bills, chores, friends, and all of modern-day life's other little demands. But many dishes on the Greek Diet take about ten minutes to make. Don't believe us? Try these recipes:

- Fish en Papillote (see page 229)
- Greek Salad (Horiatiki Salata) (see page 177)

- Greek Morning Shake (see page 284)
- Tuna Salad (Tonosalata) (see page 179)
- Watermelon Salad with Feta and Mint (see page 183)
- Baked Kale Chips (see page 278)
- Steamed Mussels (Mydia) (see page 230)
- Crunchy Toasted Chickpeas (see page 279)
- Roka Salad (see page 173)

What's more, simply making a few adjustments to your lifestyle can help you find the time it takes to make a delicious, slimming meal. Consider these tips:

- Shop for the entire week when you're at the grocery store—this habit only takes ten more minutes at most, especially if you create a shopping list before you go. Use our shopping inventory on page 21 (in the "Getting Started" section) to help you create a weekly grocery list.
- Make meals for more than one night. Depending on the size of your family, double recipes and freeze the rest so you have dinners and lunches for more than one day. Here's a list of recipes that freeze well:

  - Chicken Soup with Egg-Lemon Emulsion (Kotosoupa Avgolemono) (see page 184)
  - Wild Greens Pie (Hortopita) (see page 208)
  - Mediterranean Chicken Stew (see page 256)
  - Keftedakia (see page 247)
  - Pea and Leek Soup (Hortosoupa) (see page 185)

- Cooking is a social activity, not a chore. Invite your family or friends to help you make meals or spend time with you in the kitchen while you do.
- Use a few minutes on Sundays or before you start your workweek to cut vegetables and store them in glass containers in the fridge to use later during the week. This way, they're easy to grab and add to lunches and dinners.
- There's no rule saying you can't use precut frozen vegetables in home cooking. In fact, frozen veggies often contain more nutrients than fresh ones because they are

harvested straight from the field to the freezer, without spending a lengthy time in the open air on a truck or in a grocery store.

- A breakfast before a busy day takes only five minutes to make: Adding nuts to a bowl of Greek yogurt or scrambling eggs and veggies takes no more than five minutes— far less time than you'll spend in a brain fog at work if you go without breakfast.
- Make an extra serving of dinner during the workweek so you have something to pack for lunch the next day. Also, many dishes make easy packable lunches. Whip up one of the following recipes the day before you start your workweek and you'll have several lunches to take:

  - Lentil Salad with Oranges (see page 176)
  - Braised Giant Beans with Spinach (Gigantes me Spanaki) (see page 218)
  - Cold Red Lentil Faux Meatballs (see page 221)
  - Spanakopita Triangles (see page 206)
  - Stuffed Baby Eggplant (Papoutsakia) (see page 198)

- Salad is a quick and easy-to-pack lunch that takes no more than five minutes to make in the morning. Throw a bedding of salad greens in a glass container or screw-top jar and add precut veggies and beans as well as sliced boiled eggs; canned tuna; cooked shrimp, salmon, or chicken; or another protein source. Top with berries and a small handful of nuts. Take your salad dressing in a separate container or use olive oil spray at work.

GOING GREEK WHEN YOU'RE OUT OR ON THE GO

It's easy to stay on the Greek Diet no matter where you go, whether you want to eat out in a restaurant, have dinner at a friend's house, are traveling, get stuck in the office late, or simply don't have time to cook. Here are tips to help you stay Greek on the go:

Eating Out

Many restaurants today include some Mediterranean fare, given its popularity and addictive deliciousness. The easiest and safest option at most sit-down restaurants is some type of seafood that's not deep-fried: Look for baked, grilled, or pan-fried salmon, scallop, shrimp, tilapia, trout, bass, and other seafood dishes. Pair this with vegetables and a cooked whole grain like brown rice, farro, or quinoa if available. If not, opt for bread or a pasta with olive oil instead of butter or sugary tomato sauce. While neither of these options is likely to be whole-grain, a small serving—and keep it at small—won't sabotage your diet for one meal.

Baked, grilled, and pan-fried chicken is also a diet-friendly choice, especially if you ask for it to be cooked in olive oil with herbs and spices instead of breading, sugary sauces like barbecue, or creamy or cheesy sauces. Egg dishes can be very slimming, too, whether for breakfast or dinner—substitute feta cheese for processed cheese when possible.

Salads with fish or chicken that hasn't been breaded or fried can also be a reasonable choice if—and only if—you order carefully. Avoid bread bowls or taco shell bowls at all costs, and avoid heavy doses of processed cheese, croutons, and bacon bits—ask instead for feta cheese (a popular salad topping), beans, and/or nuts, if the dish doesn't already come with these items. Ask for olive oil and vinegar (balsamic is especially tasty) instead of traditional dressings.

Traveling or On the Go

Whether you're at the airport, on the road, or simply hungry running around doing errands on the weekend, head to a nearby travel mart, convenience store, or gas station and pick up a single-serving cup of plain Greek yogurt. Almost all stores now sell this popular snack, and when you're traveling, all you have to do is pair the yogurt with some fruit or nuts for a decent breakfast or lunch.

When you're at the office late, consider a single-serving bag of nuts (not trail mix) from the vending machine until you're able to leave for a meal. In a pinch, a small container of pretzel crisps with some hummus will do—or better yet, keep a container of hummus or yogurt with whole-grain crackers and/or carrots in the work fridge.

Ideally, though, you should aim to have meals, not snacks. So if you do have to eat at the airport, on the road, or order out from work, try to adhere to the same suggestions in the "Eating

Out" section on page 34. Many fast-food chains now offer grilled or baked chicken and seafood choices, along with healthier salads and vegetarian dishes.

WHAT IF I'M GLUTEN- OR DAIRY-FREE?

Going or staying gluten-free on the Greek Diet is simple because it includes virtually no processed foods, the majority of which contain gluten. There is also a bevy of gluten-free whole grains and whole-grain flours to cook and bake with, including brown and wild rices, quinoa, cornmeal, amaranth, buckwheat, teff, millet, and oats that specify they've been processed without gluten. Maria also has perfected the art of gluten-free cooking to help meet her clients' dietary needs at her restaurants.

Similarly, it's not difficult to avoid dairy on the Greek Diet. While you'll be forsaking one of the world's tastiest and healthiest forms of protein, Greek yogurt, you can substitute any nondairy yogurt made from soy, coconut, or almond milk that doesn't contain added sugar. But note that many of these varieties don't contain protein, so you shouldn't eat these items alone for breakfast or lunch, as they won't fill you up. Instead, choose eggs, beans, seafood, nuts, or other Pillar Foods that do contain protein.

WHAT ABOUT EXERCISE?

The reason we haven't brought up "exercise," the word most commonly associated with weight loss after "diet," until now is that we know what and how you eat is more important to losing weight than thirty minutes on a Stairmaster or a brisk walk around the neighborhood. Research has found that exercise alone can't tip the scale in the opposite direction if you're drowning yourself in the unhealthy fats, refined grains, sugar, and toxins found in most processed foods. First, it's critical you change your diet now, so that you have the energy and motivation to move, the nutrients to fuel your body when you do, and the right nutrients to help your muscles build and recover after you work out.

When you start the Greek Diet, there is no exercise prescription, no mandate that you must force yourself into a gym four times a week or go running every other day to lose weight. Instead, we want you to move as much as possible, whether that means a dedicated workout or simply adding more activity to your daily routine. This can include walking to work, taking the stairs more often, biking to run errands, playing outside with your children instead of watching TV together, going to the beach for a swim and a walk on the weekends instead of going to see a movie with friends. Don't underestimate the power of cumulative activity—studies show it can help improve your health and shrink your waistline as much as a daily trip to the gym. Remember, the ancient Greeks and other traditional cultures were able to stay lean without treadmills, Stairmasters, and exercise bikes, and we believe you can, too.

In addition to moving more, consider finding a physical activity you enjoy that increases your heart rate, and for which you can find time to do three or four times per week, such as running, walking, hiking, swimming, dancing, cycling, weight lifting, tennis, or skiing. While it's not necessary to complete dedicated workouts to lose weight, it will help you see results quicker while helping boost your mood, energy levels, and overall health. Ideally, this activity will be outdoors: Research shows people enjoy exercise more and are more likely to stick with it when they work out outside compared to inside a gym.

IS THERE ANYTHING ELSE I CAN DO TO LOSE WEIGHT?

Yes, and it's something the ancient Greeks did with gusto: Sleep. Aim to get at least six hours of sleep per night on a regular basis. Anything less than this will not only make you cranky and irritable, it will also make you hungry: Studies show inadequate sleep increases our hunger hormone, gherlin, while lowering levels of leptin, the hormone that signals our brains when we're full. What's more, research indicates that getting too little sleep boosts the tendency to binge on unhealthy foods and skip a home-cooked meal in favor of a box of cookies or bag of chips. We also move less and are less likely to exercise when we're tired.

Many people wonder whether or not if they should take dietary supplements. The short answer is no. When you adopt a healthy, balanced diet made up of primarily whole foods, your body will get all the vitamins, minerals, and antioxidants it needs. What's more, some recent research suggests multivitamins and other dietary supplements don't prevent disease and may even cause harm by interfering with liver function.

However, there are a few exceptions. Women of child-bearing age have an increased chance of developing anemia, or iron deficiency, a condition that can and will sabotage weight-loss efforts if left untreated. Additionally, vegetarians, vegans, those who take birth control pills and some other medications, and men over the age of 40 can develop less-than-ideal levels of vitamin B12, which is critical to a healthy metabolism and energy levels. If you meet any of these conditions, see a doctor who can order a blood test to see if you're deficient in iron or vitamin B12.

Finally, vegetarians, vegans, and others who don't eat seafood on a regular basis may want to consider taking a high-quality EPA/DHA supplement.

WHAT IF I DON'T SEE RESULTS?

Wait at least a week after you adopt the Greek Diet before you weigh yourself. Our bodies take time to adapt to a new eating pattern, and it's not unusual to see your body weight stuck at the same number on the scale before the needle moves in the right direction—and then, when it does, you'll usually see a big drop.

If you don't see any results after a week, chances are you're still eating the supersized amounts most Westerners have been conditioned to expect. Try following the meal plan to a T, measuring snacks and ingredients for meals for at least one week, until you have a better understanding of an appropriate portion size.

Another reason the scale could stick is if you're still eating processed foods. While it's easy to think a squirt of ketchup here or there or a cup of juice now and then won't make a difference, these extras add up over the day and certainly over the course of a week. Review our list of processed foods on pages 22–23 (in the "Getting Started" section) and try to cut every one of them out of your diet completely.

But if you're truly eating the portion sizes listed and whole foods according to the weekly menu plan and still aren't losing weight, you may have an underlying medical issue like hypothyroidism (underactive thyroid) or a nutritional deficiency like anemia, or you may be taking a medication that interferes with healthy weight loss. See your doctor for additional help and diagnosis.

MEAL PLANS
Four-Week Plan

The following four-week meal plan is based on eating 1,500 calories a day, and includes three meals, two snacks, an after-dinner snack, and a five-ounce glass of wine every day. Drink a full glass of water with every meal and snack, or, alternatively, between meals and snacks.

FOUR-WEEK MEAL PLAN

WEEK 1

Asterisk indicates recipe included.

	Breakfast	Mid-Morning Snack	Lunch	Afternoon Snack	Dinner	Dessert/ Evening Snack
SUNDAY	Greek Frittata* AND Coffee or tea	1 orange	Baked Salmon with Yogurt Sauce* AND Marouli Salad with Feta-Yogurt Dressing*	Crunchy Toasted Chickpeas*	Baked Shrimp with Feta Cheese in Tomato Sauce (Saganaki Shrimp)* AND 5 oz. wine	Greek mountain tea
					TOTAL: 1,500 calories, 61 grams protein	
MONDAY	1 bowl oatmeal made with ¼ cup dry steel cut oats and water, topped with ½ cup fresh sliced peaches and ¼ cup chopped walnuts AND Coffee or tea	2 small plums	Couscous Salad*	Baked Apple Chips*	Grilled Chicken Breast* AND Braised Green Beans (Fasolakia)* OR Any grilled chicken breast and side salad or side of braised, steamed, or grilled vegetables AND 5 oz. wine	1 cup blackberries
					TOTAL: 1,600 calories, 69 grams protein	
TUESDAY	Greek Morning Shake* (includes coffee)	1 cup blueberries	Lentil Salad with Oranges*	1 cup 2% plain Greek yogurt	Salmon with Fennel and Leeks* AND 5 oz. wine	1 cup cherries
					TOTAL: 1,500 calories, 81 grams protein	
WEDNESDAY	Scrambled Eggs with Feta Cheese (Kayana)* AND Coffee or tea	1 medium apple	Lentil Soup (Fakes)* OR Cannellini Bean Soup (Fasolada)* OR Takeout bowl of bean-based soup	¼ cup Maria's Hummus* with celery stalks	Artichoke Stew with vegetables* AND 5 oz. wine	1 cup Frozen Greek Yogurt* AND Greek mountain tea
					TOTAL: 1,500 calories, 78 grams protein	

	Breakfast	Mid-Morning Snack	Lunch	Afternoon Snack	Dinner	Dessert/ Evening Snack
THURSDAY	1 cup 2% plain Greek yogurt AND 1 cup strawberries AND Coffee or tea	1 medium peach	Pomegranate Kale Salad* AND Cold Red Lentil Faux Meatballs*	Greek mountain tea	Fish en Papillote* AND Braised Green Beans (Fasolakia Lemonata)* OR Any grilled, broiled, steamed, poached, or baked fish (about the size of the palm of your hand) and a side salad or side of braised, steamed, or grilled vegetables AND 5 oz. wine	Greek mountain tea
					TOTAL: 1,600 calories, 64 grams protein	
FRIDAY	Greek Morning Shake* (includes coffee)	1 small apple	Lentil Soup (Fakes)*	2 small plums	Chicken and Mushroom Souvlaki* AND Couscous Salad* AND 5 oz. wine	1 cup blueberries
					TOTAL: 1,500 calories, 62 grams protein	
SATURDAY	1 cup 2% plain Greek yogurt topped with ½ cup fresh blackberries AND Coffee or tea	1 cup grapes	Vegetarian Moussaka* OR Braised Giant Beans with Spinach (Gigantes Me Spanaki)* OR Any bean-based dish with leafy greens	½ cup pistachios with shells	Watermelon Salad with Feta and Mint* AND Salmon Souvlaki* AND 5 oz. wine	Rice Pudding (Rizogalo)*
					TOTAL: 1,500 calories, 76 grams protein	

WEEK 2

	Breakfast	Mid-Morning Snack	Lunch	Afternoon Snack	Dinner	Dessert/ Evening Snack
SUNDAY	Greek Frittata* AND Coffee or tea	½ cup strawberries and ½ cup blueberries	Pumpkin and Zucchini Pie (Kolokithopita)*	1 cup raspberries	Spring Stuffed Leg of Lamb (Boutaki Yemisto)* AND 5 oz. wine	1 medium peach AND Greek mountain tea
					TOTAL: 1,400 calories, 93 grams protein	
MONDAY	Oatmeal made with ¼ cup steel cut oats and water, topped with ½ cup blueberries AND Coffee or tea	1 medium banana	Lentil Soup (Fakes)*	Crunchy Toasted Chickpeas*	Vegetable Stew (Turlu)* OR Any broth-based vegetable soup AND 5 oz. wine	Rice Pudding (Rizogalo)* AND Greek mountain tea
					TOTAL: 1,500 calories, 57 grams protein	
TUESDAY	Scrambled Eggs with Feta Cheese (Kayana)* AND Coffee or tea	1 medium peach	Tahini Vegetable Soup (Tahinosoupa)* AND Grilled Chicken Breast*	1 cup raspberries	Artichokes with Rice and Vegetables* AND 5 oz. wine	1 cup Frozen Greek Yogurt*
					TOTAL: 1,500 calories, 94 grams protein	
WEDNESDAY	Greek Morning Shake* (includes coffee)	1 cup raspberries	Lentil Salad with Oranges*	1 cup cubed cantaloupe	Steamed Mussels (Mydia)* AND 5 oz. wine	Greek mountain tea
					TOTAL: 1,500 calories, 82 grams protein	

	Breakfast	Mid-Morning Snack	Lunch	Afternoon Snack	Dinner	Dessert/ Evening Snack
THURSDAY	¾ cup 2% plain Greek yogurt with ½ cup strawberries AND 1 cup raspberries AND Coffee or tea	1 medium pear	Watermelon Salad with Feta and Mint* AND Grilled Chicken Breast*	1 medium peach	Braised Cauliflower (Kounoupidi)* AND Spaghetti with Fresh Tomato Sauce* AND 5 oz. wine	1 cup cherries AND Greek mountain tea

TOTAL: 1,600 calories, 85 grams protein

	Breakfast	Mid-Morning Snack	Lunch	Afternoon Snack	Dinner	Dessert/ Evening Snack
FRIDAY	Greek Morning Shake* (includes coffee)	1 cup cubed cantaloupe	Greek Salad (Horiatiki Salata)* with Cucumber Dressing* OR Takeout Greek salad	1 cup 2% plain Greek yogurt topped with ½ cup blackberries	Wheat Berry Salad* OR Any leafy green–based salad with nuts, beans, or seeds AND 5 oz. wine	1 cup blueberries

TOTAL: 1,500 calories, 58 grams protein

	Breakfast	Mid-Morning Snack	Lunch	Afternoon Snack	Dinner	Dessert/ Evening Snack
SATURDAY	Oatmeal made with ¼ cup steel cut oats and water, topped with ½ cup blueberries AND Coffee or tea	1 cup strawberries	Zucchini Croquettes (Kolokithokeftedes)* with ½ cup Roasted Beet–Yogurt Dip*	½ cup 2% plain Greek yogurt topped with ½ cup blueberries	Fish en Papillote* AND Braised Green Beans (Fasolakia Lemonata)* AND 5 oz. wine	Greek Baked Apples*

TOTAL: 1,600 calories, 60 grams protein

WEEK 3

	Breakfast	Mid-Morning Snack	Lunch	Afternoon Snack	Dinner	Dessert/ Evening Snack
SUNDAY	Greek Frittata* AND 1 cup cubed cantaloupe AND Coffee or tea	1 cup strawberries	Stuffed Zucchini (Zucchini Gemista)*	1 medium peach	Lean Beef Patties with Oats (Keftedakia)* AND Braised Green Beans (Fasolakia)* AND 5 oz. wine	Greek mountain tea
					TOTAL: 1,500 calories, 66 grams protein	
MONDAY	Oatmeal made with ¼ cup steel cut oats and water, topped with ½ cup blueberries AND Coffee or tea	1 medium peach	1 cup 2% plain Greek yogurt topped with ½ oz. (7 halves) chopped walnuts and 1 tsp. honey	1 cup raspberries	Tuna Salad (Tonosalata)* AND 5 oz. wine	Rice Pudding (Rizogalo)*
					TOTAL: 1,500 calories, 78 grams protein	
TUESDAY	Greek Morning Shake* (includes coffee)	1 cup raspberries	Lentil Soup (Fakes)*	Baked Apple Chips*	Greek Salad (Horiatiki Salata)* with Cucumber Dressing* AND Grilled Chicken Breast* AND 5 oz. wine	1 medium peach
					TOTAL: 1,500 calories, 79 grams protein	
WEDNESDAY	Scrambled Eggs with Feta Cheese (Kayana)* AND Coffee or tea	½ cup 2% plain Greek yogurt topped with ½ cup blackberries	Couscous Salad*	¼ cup Maria's Hummus* with celery stalks	Quinoa Pilafaki with Shrimp, Lemon, and Herbs* AND 5 oz. wine	1 cup cherries
					TOTAL: 1,500 calories, 71 grams protein	

	Breakfast	Mid-Morning Snack	Lunch	Afternoon Snack	Dinner	Dessert/ Evening Snack
THURSDAY	Oatmeal made with ¼ cup steel cut oats and water, topped with 1 medium peach, sliced, AND Coffee or tea	1 medium banana	Pomegranate Kale Salad* AND ½ cup 2% plain Greek yogurt topped with 1 tsp. honey	1 oz. pistachios	Grilled Chicken Breast* AND Mushroom Barley Soup* AND 5 oz. wine	1 cup raspberries

TOTAL: 1,600 calories, 72 grams protein

	Breakfast	Mid-Morning Snack	Lunch	Afternoon Snack	Dinner	Dessert/ Evening Snack
FRIDAY	Greek Morning Shake* (includes Greek coffee) AND 1 cup raspberries	¾ cup 2% plain Greek yogurt topped with ½ cup strawberries and ½ oz. almonds	Marouli Salad with Feta-Yogurt Dressing*	Crunchy Toasted Chickpeas*	Artichokes with Rice and Vegetables* AND 5 oz. wine	1 cup blackberries

TOTAL: 1,500 calories, 63 grams protein

	Breakfast	Mid-Morning Snack	Lunch	Afternoon Snack	Dinner	Dessert/ Evening Snack
SATURDAY	1 cup 2% plain Greek yogurt topped with ½ cup blueberries AND Coffee or tea	1 cup cherries	Chicken and Mushroom Souvlaki* AND Mashed Cauliflower with Roasted Garlic*	Baked Kale Chips*	Bulgur Pilafaki with Mussels* AND 5 oz. wine	1 Almond Cookie (Amigdalota)* AND Greek mountain tea

TOTAL: 1,500 calories, 78 grams protein

WEEK 4

	Breakfast	Mid-Morning Snack	Lunch	Afternoon Snack	Dinner	Dessert/ Evening Snack
SUNDAY	Greek Frittata* AND Coffee or tea	1 cup cubed cantaloupe	Baked Salmon with Yogurt Sauce* AND Marouli Salad with Feta-Yogurt Dressing*	1 cup strawberries	Mediterranean Chicken Stew* AND 5 oz. wine	Greek mountain tea
					TOTAL: 1,500 calories, 75 grams protein	
MONDAY	1 cup 2% plain Greek yogurt topped with 1 medium banana, sliced AND Coffee or tea	1 oz. walnuts (about 1 handful or 14 halves)	Lentil Salad with Oranges*	1 medium pear	Artichokes with Rice and Vegetables* AND 5 oz. wine	Greek mountain tea
					TOTAL: 1,600 calories, 64 grams protein	
TUESDAY	Oatmeal made with ¼ cup steel cut oats and water, topped with ⅛ cup of chopped walnuts and sprinkled with cinnamon AND Coffee or tea	1 cup blackberries	Couscous Salad* OR Any salad made with mixed vegetables with 1 serving of beans, nuts, and/or grilled chicken or shrimp	Crunchy Toasted Chickpeas*	Marouli Salad with Feta-Yogurt Dressing* AND Grilled Chicken Breast* AND 5 oz. wine	1 cup cubed cantaloupe
					TOTAL: 1,500 calories, 72 grams protein	

	Breakfast	Mid-Morning Snack	Lunch	Afternoon Snack	Dinner	Dessert/ Evening Snack
WEDNESDAY	Scrambled Eggs with Feta Cheese (Kayana)* AND Coffee or tea	1 medium peach	Marouli Salad with Feta-Yogurt Dressing* AND Grilled Chicken Breast*	1 medium orange	Bulgur Pilafaki with Mussels* OR Any grilled shrimp or other fish (about the size of the palm of your hand) with a side salad and a baked sweet potato or a side of quinoa, brown rice, or other whole grain AND 5 oz. wine	1 cup cherries
					TOTAL: 1,500 calories, 76 grams protein	
THURSDAY	Greek Morning Shake* (includes coffee)	1 cup raspberries	Watermelon Salad with Feta and Mint* AND Greek Frittata*	½ cup pistachios	Fish en Papillote* AND Braised Green Beans (Fasolakia Lemonata)* AND 5 oz. wine	1 slice Carrot Cake* (only made with Maria's recipe) AND Greek mountain tea
					TOTAL: 1,500 calories, 66 grams protein	
FRIDAY	Oatmeal made with ¼ cup steel cut oats and water, topped with ½ cup blueberries and ½ cup strawberries AND Coffee or tea	1 cup 2% plain Greek yogurt	Lentil Soup (Fakes)* AND Vegetable Souvlaki*	1 medium peach	Vegetable Stew (Turlu)* AND 5 oz. wine	Greek mountain tea
					TOTAL: 1,500 calories, 71 grams protein	

	Breakfast	Mid-Morning Snack	Lunch	Afternoon Snack	Dinner	Dessert/ Evening Snack
SATURDAY	Scrambled Eggs with Feta Cheese (Kayana)* OR Any egg dish made with 2 eggs and 1 slice of cheese AND Coffee or tea	Fruit salad made with 1 medium peach and 1 cup blueberries	Grilled Branzino with Tomato-Kalamata Tapenade*	½ cup 2% plain Greek yogurt topped with ½ cup blackberries	Vegetarian Moussaka* AND 5 oz. wine	Rice Pudding (Rizogalo)* with ½ cup raspberries

TOTAL: 1,500 calories, 76 grams protein

PART III

THE TWELVE PILLAR FOODS

Pillar One:	Olive Oil		Pillar Seven:	Wine
Pillar Two:	Yogurt		Pillar Eight:	Herbs and Spices
Pillar Three:	Vegetables		Pillar Nine:	Fruit
Pillar Four:	Beans		Pillar Ten:	Coffee and Tea
Pillar Five:	Seafood		Pillar Eleven:	Nuts and Seeds
Pillar Six:	Whole Grains		Pillar Twelve:	Chicken and Eggs

Supplemental Foods

Olive Oil (Sensual)

I NEVER KNEW olive oil was the secret to losing weight until I was in my forties and already overweight. That's when I met Dr. Joseph Nikolaides. He and his wife were on vacation from Athens in my village of Nafpaktos, home to my restaurant Kouzina Maria Loi. When I first met him I didn't know he was a doctor. I saw only a fit man and a beautiful woman eating many, many plates of food—fish, chicken, salad, bread, even dessert!

Eventually, I couldn't stand it. One day, I asked them how they stayed so thin. The doctor's answer was simple: First he told me he never used butter—he consumed only olive oil, no other vegetable oils or fats. He said he was careful about what he put in his body, comparing himself to an expensive vehicle, putting only the best gas in. He said he ate the same foods he grew up on, enjoying a traditional, healthy Greek diet.

At first I was surprised, and then I got so mad! Why did I stop eating the foods I grew up on? It had started in my thirties, when my career as a successful lobbyist for big multinational corporations took off. I was traveling more, and snacking more, eating more Americanized foods—fast food at airports, packaged snacks like chips, and, I am ashamed to say it, butter on everything. Butter! I had never eaten butter in my life! In two and a half years, I had gained forty pounds! I tried dieting and would lose a few pounds, but then it would come back—I felt awful. I started to eat less and less, but the only change was that I kept gaining more and more.

A decade later, nothing had changed—I was still carrying those extra forty pounds. I told Dr. Nikolaides about my diet and weight troubles—he told me the first thing I should do was stop eating butter and other fats, and start eating olive oil, and so I did.

Within several weeks, I had lost 10 pounds—I couldn't believe it! I was eating the same amount and types of food—the only difference was that I put olive oil in my mouth, too. It felt wonderful, like my whole body—my face, my stomach, my hips—was deflating.

After a few weeks on my olive oil diet, I noticed I wasn't as hungry as often. When I ate bread, one slice was enough. My salads needed less dressing. I didn't even care if I ate dessert. And I wasn't even trying to eat less! But the olive oil was keeping me full, balancing my body and giving it the healthy fat I had been craving for years.

While I was happy with my weight loss, I was also frustrated with myself. I had known my whole life that olive oil was a health-giving, satisfying, and essential food. My family raised our own olive trees, and every year, we made our own oil. Our olive trees were beautiful and healthy, and our olive oil was the best in our village. To me as a child, olive oil wasn't just a food—it was one of my first loves.

GROWING UP ON OLIVE OIL

My earliest memory growing up was the smell of our house. It smelled like olive oil. The fragrance came from our cellar, where my family stored our barrels of olive oil. We were poor, but we had acres of land, where we raised over 500 olive trees. These trees were like my toys, the only things my parents could afford for me and my brother and sisters to play with.

When I was a young girl, I planted over 100 trees with my father—and I took care of them. I pruned them, picked off their rotting olives, watered them, and shaded them when the sun got too hot. I loved my trees. Even today, when I go back home, I can still pick out the trees I planted (olive trees live for hundreds of years)—these are my favorite trees, the ones I remember loving as a child.

From all my family's olive trees, we made olive oil. Every fall, everyone—my father, mother, three sisters, brother, and grandparents, along with friends from our village—would go out into the fields and gather the olives, shaking the trees and handpicking the best fruit. We would put all the olives we chose in a special bag so they wouldn't become bruised, and then walk them to the *eleotrivio,* a big wooden olive press in the middle of our village. This was special—not every village had an eleotrivio. Ours was operated by donkeys, which pulled a long wooden beam that extended from the center of the press in a large circle. This drove a stone grinder that crushed the olives and sent their juice running out into a big metal pot.

The juice from the eleotrivio was unlike anything else: The first press came out as a beautiful green color, rich and thick, and the fragrance reminded me of freshly cut grass. And it tasted like heaven. I always went to the eleotrivio with a cup in my pocket and some fresh bread my grandmother or mother had baked that morning, so I could taste the first press. I was the youngest, so I was allowed to sneak to the front of the line. I remember feeling so lucky while eating my bread with the first drippings from the press. After I ate, I would take a couple of drops of oil in my hands and rub them together so I could smell the fruitiness from the olives all day long, the way my grandfather had taught me.

At home, my family ate olive oil at every meal, even dessert. In the morning, we drizzled olive oil over our eggs and dipped our fresh bread in it. For lunch, our main meal of the day, everything we ate was cooked in olive oil—our tomatoes, fish, and beans. In the afternoon, if we wanted to eat something, we dipped a piece of bread in olive oil. Dinner was smaller than our lunch, and we often had leftovers, but my favorite dinner was when my parents allowed us to grill our bread in the fireplace, and we'd then soak it in olive oil. For dessert, my mother and grandmother would make *melomakarona,* an olive-oil cookie dipped in honey. But even when I was very young, I liked to make my own desserts. I used to pour olive oil on my hands, and then mash soft bread into an olive oil–soaked dough ball. I would then roll these little olive-oil treats in honey, and then crushed nuts or cinnamon.

As I was growing up, my family didn't just eat olive oil, we also used it as medicine. In America, people say, "An apple a day keeps the doctor away," but in Greece, we say a couple of tablespoons of olive oil a day will keep *many* doctors away. My grandfather used to give all of us children one tablespoon of olive oil every morning after we woke up. This was a tradition in our family for generations; instead of vitamins, you took olive oil. We loved to drink the oil off his spoon—we would line up like little chickens waiting for our feed. My grandfather told us if we drank it every day, our hair and eyes would shine, we would have better teeth, and we would be healthier. And he was right: A few of my friends in my village who didn't drink olive oil never looked as healthy as we did.

My oldest sister and I also used olive oil as a beauty aid. We would coat our hair in it weekly, leaving the oil in all day and overnight until we bathed again, which made our hair so soft and smell so fruity. My middle sisters thought it was strange and didn't do it, and they never had hair as thick or beautiful as my oldest sister's or mine. As I grew older, I also dabbed olive oil around my eyes at night when I was tired, so I wouldn't wake up with black circles. I still do that today!

A Better (and Cheaper!) Hair Conditioner

WHAT WE NEED

2 tablespoons olive oil

¼ cup of Greek yogurt

Few drops of an essential oil like lavender, lemon, rose, or mint (optional)

WHAT WE DO

Mix the oil and yogurt together in a bowl. Massage into wet hair, coating from root to tip. If your hair is long, clip it up or use a shower cap, then lounge for 30 minutes, letting your hair absorb the mixture. Rinse thoroughly in warm water and look forward to fuller, thicker, and shinier hair.

OLIVE OIL IN ANCIENT GREECE

When I was growing up, everyone in my village ate olive oil. No one even had butter, canola oil, lard, or anything else in their houses. On every table in every home at every meal, you could always find a bottle of olive oil. And it had been like this for centuries.

The ancient Greeks were the first to cultivate olive trees and use them to make olive oil. This was an essential staple of the ancient Greek diet. They ate a lot of bread, and all that bread would get dipped in olive oil. They would marinate their fish and meat in olive oil, then wrap it in fig leaves before cooking it. They would add olive oil to their beans and vegetables after they cooked them, for flavor. Like my family, they also believed olive oil had medicinal powers and fed it to their sick and healthy alike. They used the oil as a moisturizer and salve, rubbing it all over their bodies every day.

In ancient Greek mythology, olive oil was symbolic, a sacred gift. It's also how the city of Athens got its name. According to the myth, Athena, the goddess of wisdom, got into a competition with Poseidon, the Greek god of the sea and horses. Both gods wanted to be the one to name the capital of Greece, a new city growing in the heart of the country. In order to decide who would name their city, the citizens wanted a useful gift from each god. Poseidon gave them warhorses and pierced his trident into the land, causing seawater to spring up. Athena responded by striking a rock with her spear, causing an olive tree to grow there. It didn't take the citizens long to decide who had won: They knew the olive tree would bring them good health and flavorful food year round, from olives and olive oil. The city declared Athena had won and chose the name of Athens for itself. Today, Athens continues to be the country's cultural and governmental epicenter.

Olive Oil for Dry, Brittle Nails

WHAT WE NEED

1 tablespoon olive oil
1 teaspoon lemon juice

WHAT WE DO

Microwave the olive oil in a small bowl until just warm (approximately ten seconds), being careful not to overheat the oil. Add the lemon juice. Before bed, soak your nails in the mixture for 20 minutes. Then, slip your hands into a pair of inexpensive fabric gloves (you can find these at many supermarkets, pharmacies, and dollar stores) and wake up with stronger, healthier nails!

OLIVE OIL TODAY

Olive oil is the only oil—or fat of any kind—I use. At my restaurants, we have no butter, lard, canola oil, peanut oil, corn oil, or any other fats in our kitchen. I use only olive oil, not just because I grew up on it, but also because I believe it's the healthiest fat and one of the healthiest ingredients in the world. Olive oil helps lower your cholesterol and blood pressure, it fights heart disease, it keeps your insulin levels balanced, and it supplies your body with the healthy fat you need to live, be happy, and be thin.

Olive oil isn't just the healthiest oil, it is also the tastiest oil! As a chef, I learned years ago that the fat you use to cook with determines how your food tastes. For example, when you cook green beans in butter, you taste only the butter. But when you cook green beans in olive oil, you can taste the earthy freshness of the green beans, and it's beautiful. It's how food should taste— pure and fresh. Over time, you start to crave the beans for how they taste, not for the fat they're cooked in. Since this is true of all good-for-you ingredients—other vegetables, fish, bread— making food with olive oil can help you become a healthier eater, not because you're trying, but because it makes you want to eat these foods.

In this sense, olive oil is one of the world's ultimate pleasure foods. It overwhelms your senses: The flavor is fruity yet spicy all at the same time, the texture feels thick and rich in your mouth, and the smell is aromatic and intoxicating. Whenever I eat olive oil, I feel it moving through every nerve ending in my body, as if the olive oil is saying, "Here I am, it's me, olive oil!" Whenever I feel tired or down, I drink one or two tablespoons. I don't take medicines, have energy drinks, or use antidepressants—I just eat more olive oil. It's like a drug. It gets in your veins!

I feel so strongly about olive oil—and tell everyone I know to use it—that the Greek Association of Industries and Processors of Olive Oil, known as Sevitel, asked me several years ago to be the Greek Ambassador of Olive Oil. In my role today, I teach people how to cook and use olive oil in the most healthy, flavorful ways possible. I appear regularly on major network television shows like *Good Morning America* and at international culinary events like the Aspen Food & Wine Festival. I also hold cooking classes and demonstrations at nonprofit organizations around the country, educating people on the merits of olive oil.

Extra-Virgin, Virgin, Pure . . . What's the Difference?

Most people are familiar with extra-virgin olive oil, but if you head to the store, you'll find dozens of different types of olive oil. For most cooking purposes, we prefer extra-virgin olive oil (EVOO) and virgin olive oil (VOO): Both are low in acid and unrefined, meaning they're pressed in the traditional way and not chemically processed after the pressing. Here's how the five most common commercial olive oils stack up in terms of smoke point (the temperature at which they begin to break down), best uses, and flavor:

TYPE	DEFINITION	SMOKE POINT	BEST USES	FLAVOR
Extra-virgin	Made from first cold pressing	375–405°F	Dips, dressings, drizzlings, garnishing, some sautéing, and other cold uses	Fruity, earthy, peppery, grassy, buttery, and fragrant
Virgin	Made from second cold pressing	390°F	Medium-heat sautéing and pan-frying	Less fruity and rich than EVOO, but still has a distinct olive taste

Pure	Made from second cold pressing or chemical extraction	410°F	Roasting, baking, and deep-frying (if you have to)	Not as strong or fragrant as EVOO or VOO
Light	A combo of virgin oil and refined oils, not lower in fat or calories	470°F	Avoid if possible. Lacks health benefits.	Nearly tasteless, with a slight olive aftertaste. No fragrance.
Pomace	A combo of leftover batches of virgin and refined oils	460°F	Avoid by all means. Low-quality oil that lacks health benefits.	Bitter and dingy olive taste and fragrance

HOW I USE OLIVE OIL

The question shouldn't be "What do you use olive oil for?"—it should be "What *don't* you use olive oil for?" Any time we want to add fat to food, we use olive oil. This includes grilling, marinating, pan-frying, searing, and even baking. If you eat at my restaurants, your meal starts with some fresh pita bread and a small dish of extra-virgin olive oil. All of our dressings, traditional Greek spreads, and sauces are made with olive oil, and we drizzle it over cold and cooked plates of vegetables. When you order an entrée like fish or meat, it was marinated or cooked in olive oil. We use olive oil instead of butter to moisten phyllo dough when we make spanakopita and other Greek pies. Half of our desserts are made with olive oil, like walnut cake, apple pie, and baklava. For our customers who want more American-style desserts, we serve cakes made with an olive-oil margarine.

But just because olive oil is healthy, it doesn't mean I drown my food in it. Quite the opposite—we actually use less olive oil than at many other Mediterranean restaurants. This helps our customers taste our fresh ingredients, herbs, and spices—not just the fat the food was cooked or dressed in. But it also helps keep you healthy—any food that's too oily or fatty is not good for you. The ancient Greek philosophers believed strongly in *metron ariston*, "everything in moderation," and that is how I was raised, too.

Today, I cook differently with olive oil than my family did growing up. When I was little, my parents and grandparents would put oil in every pan before they cooked, whether it was fish, beans, or greens. While there is nothing wrong with cooking food this way, I found if you wait until a food is almost done cooking to add the olive oil to the pan, you don't need to use as much. The natural flavor of your ingredients is also stronger and more exciting for your taste buds. This is what makes the Greek Diet different—everyone knows olive oil is good for you, but few people know how to use it properly to make healthy food taste so wonderful.

When I add olive oil to cold foods or ones that have already been cooked, I use only extra-virgin olive oil (EVOO). EVOO has a fruitier taste than other types of olive oil, and I believe it brings more satisfaction to your mouth and palate. Also, when you use EVOO, you don't have to use as much olive oil because it's higher quality and the texture and taste are richer and more flavorful. For example, when I make hummus, I use extra-virgin olive oil. This gives the hummus a pleasant, smoother, richer taste and lets me savor the other ingredients in the hummus, including the chickpeas, lemon, herbs, and spices, not just the oil. It's also healthier than many store-bought brands of hummus. (See page 270 for the recipe.)

So how much olive oil should you eat a day on the Greek Diet? We tell people to try to get 3 to 4 tablespoons a day. You don't need to count, but it helps to pay attention to how much you use in cooking, salad dressings, dips, and other foods. Our recipes and meal plans are specially designed to help you maintain the right balance of olive oil with other foods and fats. But, even if you don't have time to make home-cooked meals every day, simply asking for your food to be cooked in olive oil at restaurants can help you lose weight, feel fuller, and stay happy and healthy for life.

Common Cooking Oils and Smoke Points

It's important to know the smoke point of any fat or oil you're cooking with because once it starts to break down, the flavor, texture, and overall character of the oil are compromised—and all the health benefits attributed to that fat or oil are negated. In fact, any fat or oil heated past its smoke point can have harmful effects, including increasing your risk for cancer.

FATS/OILS	SMOKE POINT	IDEAL HEAT FOR COOKING PURPOSES
Clarified butter	485°F	High
Butter	300°F	Low
Canola	400°F	Medium to High
Corn	450°F	High
Coconut	350°F	Low to Medium
Grapeseed	485°F	High
Olive	375–465°F	Medium to High
Peanut	450°F	High
Soybean	450°F	High
Vegetable	Variable	Variable

PILLAR ONE
Olive Oil (Science)

YOU DON'T HAVE TO EAT LESS, exercise more, or count calories or carbs to start your weight-loss journey—you simply have to consume more olive oil. That's the take home from dozens of studies showing that substituting olive oil for other fats in your diet can help your body burn fat, curb your appetite, increase your metabolism, and trigger weight loss. In fact, some studies have even found that people who ate olive oil *ad libitum,* meaning as much as they wanted, still lost body fat. How can olive oil, high in both fat and calories, be a fat-burning food? Here are the top three ways olive oil will turn your body into a fat-burning machine:

1. OLIVE OIL CONTAINS THE KIND OF FAT YOUR BODY NEEDS TO BURN FAT.

Not all fats are created equal when it comes to how they affect our bodies. Some fats can cause us to gain weight, while others are absolutely essential to helping our bodies burn fat. Perhaps the most important fat for weight loss is monounsaturated fat, or MUFA. Olive oil contains more MUFA than almost any other common oil or food. Olive oil is made up of 75 percent MUFA— by comparison, soybean oil, used in many packaged foods, has only 23 percent MUFA, while butter contains 29 percent (the rest is mostly saturated fat).

Research has found that eating more MUFA helps your body lose weight in a variety of ways. First, MUFA forces your body to burn fat without you doing anything at all. A study conducted in Australia found that eating a breakfast high in MUFA (think olive oil on toast, in eggs, or over yogurt—or a spoonful of olive oil in the morning, like Maria's grandfather gave her) increases fat oxidization, or the body's ability to use fat as a fuel source. This applies to every food you eat during the day: If you add MUFA to your meals and snacks, you'll bump up your body's ability to burn fat. Second, studies have found that consuming MUFA-rich olive oil instead of foods high in saturated fat significantly increases your resting energy expenditure, or the amount of energy your body uses at rest. This means your body will burn more calories when sitting, driving, eating, or just sleeping.

Olive oil is not only exceedingly high in MUFA, it's also high in a type of MUFA called oleic acid—in fact, oleic acid is the main component in olive oil. Recently, oleic acid has become a hot-button topic in the weight-loss world. A groundbreaking study found that when people consume high amounts of oleic acid, it gets converted into a hormone called oleoylethanolamide that helps stop hunger pangs and increases the feelings of fullness between meals. In addition, oleic acid has been shown to lower blood-sugar levels and help control insulin, one of your body's fat-storing hormones.

2. OLIVE OIL IS SUCH A POWERFUL WEIGHT-LOSS STIMULANT, EVEN THE SMELL CAN HELP YOU SHED POUNDS.

Olive oil has certain unique properties that trigger weight loss in ways other foods high in MUFA and oleic acid do not (although olive oil is one of the highest dietary sources of both). A groundbreaking study from Germany surprised nutritionists worldwide when it discovered that the scent of olive oil helps people feel fuller and instinctively eat fewer calories throughout the day. Researchers recruited over 120 people, divided them into groups, and fed them plain yogurt or yogurt mixed either with olive oil, canola oil, butter, or lard. After months of study, the researchers discovered that those who were eating the olive-oil yogurt had much higher levels of serotonin, a hormone that increases feelings of fullness and happiness. The olive-oil group also consumed fewer calories during the day than the other three groups, compensating without realizing it for the extra calories in the yogurt. By comparison, those who ate yogurt with canola oil—which contains a high level of MUFA, too—didn't experience any increase in serotonin, ate more calories throughout the day, and ended up gaining weight over the three-month study!

Shocked by the results, the researchers repeated the study, but instead of adding olive oil to yogurt, they stirred in a grassy scent extract from the aromatic oil. True enough, the same effect occurred: Those who ate yogurt scented with olive oil had higher serotonin levels, ate fewer calories, and had better blood-sugar levels after the meal. The researchers concluded that simply the scent of olive oil—the fruity, grassy aroma Maria and the ancient Greeks grew up inhaling—is a potent weight-loss aid that can help people feel fuller and happier in a matter of moments.

3. INCREASING YOUR INTAKE OF OLIVE OIL WILL BOOST YOUR OVERALL HEALTH, HELPING SPEED YOUR WEIGHT LOSS.

By now, most people know that olive oil is one of the heart-healthiest foods on the face of the planet, capable of lowering LDL ("bad") cholesterol, fighting high blood pressure, and reducing your overall risk of heart disease—the number one killer in the United States. A large-scale study of nearly 41,000 adults in 2012 found that consuming just 2 tablespoons of olive oil every day cuts your risk of dying of heart disease in half! In 2013, a rigorously undertaken study of over 7,400 people in Spain found that eating a Mediterranean diet high in olive oil reduced the risk of having a heart attack or stroke by up to 30 percent. Doctors who analyzed the research concluded that eating an olive oil–rich Mediterranean diet had similar effects to taking statins, the popular cholesterol-lowering drugs used by one in four Americans over the age of 45.

The Spanish research isn't the only study to show olive oil is as effective at controlling risk factors of heart disease as taking prescription drugs (many of which, like statins, have undesirable side effects, including muscle pain, liver damage, and yikes!, a rise in the weight-gaining hormone insulin). For example, one study shows that replacing 40 percent of the saturated fat in your diet (from butter, cream, and other oils) with olive oil can reduce your LDL cholesterol by as much as 15 percent. As to blood pressure, Italian researchers found that consuming 4 tablespoons of olive oil per day—the same daily dose recommended on the Greek Diet—can reduce the need for blood pressure medication by 50 percent.

Part of olive oil's heart-healthy effects extend from the same fat that triggers weight loss: MUFA. Monounsaturated fatty acids have been shown to reduce LDL cholesterol (without reducing HDL, or "good," cholesterol), lower chronic inflammation throughout the body, and stabilize heart rhythms. But there's more to it than just MUFA: Unlike butter and many other oils, olive oil, especially extra-virgin and virgin, is very high in antioxidants, particularly a powerful class of antioxidants called polyphenols. These antioxidants, also found in wine and dark chocolate, have been shown to combat inflammation and protect blood vessels on a genetic level.

But olive oil's health benefits extend far beyond your heart and cardiovascular system. Olive oil is one of the longest and most rigorously studied health foods in the world, and now a multitude of studies have found increasing your intake of olive oil can reduce many types of cancer, including breast, lung, stomach, and, to a lesser extent, colorectal cancer. For women on the Greek Diet, the effect is pronounced: Three out of five Cornell University studies show consuming a high amount of olive oil specifically causes a significant decrease in the risk of breast cancer.

And the list goes on: Olive oil has also been shown to reduce blood-sugar levels, which not only helps you lose weight, but also prevents diabetes—a growing epidemic in America that is quickly affecting more and more people. Olive oil also helps prevent digestive problems by slowing the growth of unwanted bacteria and protecting the stomach lining from ulcers and other complications. And milk isn't the only food that can do a body good: Research strongly suggests olive oil can increase calcium levels and bone formation. Finally, large-scale studies show high intakes of the oil improve brain health, preventing certain diseases like Alzheimer's, while increasing memory, verbal skills, and other cognitive functions.

PILLAR TWO
Yogurt (Sensual)

GREEK YOGURT IS ONE OF THE RICHEST, creamiest, most filling, and most satisfying foods you can eat. The ancient Greeks knew how delicious it was—they invented it! Now, thousands of years later, nutritionists are finally realizing how valuable this fantastic food is for helping people stay thin, strong, and healthy. I eat it every day and have done so for years. Greek yogurt is packed with protein to help fill you up—double the amount in regular American yogurt—and is full of healthy bacteria called probiotics to feed your metabolism and digestive system so fat can just melt away.

Protein and probiotics make Greek yogurt a great diet food, but its taste and texture make it fantastic! Thick, creamy, and rich, Greek yogurt is one of the world's ultimate pleasure foods. That it also happens to be good for you and helps you lose weight is why it's central to the Greek Diet. After I have a cup of Greek yogurt, I don't want any other food—my stomach is full, and I feel stronger, healthier, and more energetic. Some people drink sugary sodas or eat sweets to pick themselves up—I eat yogurt!

For these reasons, I eat yogurt every day. In the morning, I like my yogurt with a little honey or fruit—one or the other, not both, to keep my sugar levels low. If I have cereal, I make muesli with yogurt, not milk, because milk makes me puffy (yogurt makes me happy). When I have an omelet or *frutalia* (Greek frittata), I add yogurt to the eggs before I cook them, which makes them fluffier and creamier. I also like to eat my eggs with a dollop of yogurt on top—delicious! For lunch and dinner, I dress salads with yogurt mixed with a little olive oil and feta cheese. Instead of mayonnaise, I spread yogurt on sandwiches and use it in chicken and potato salad. For me, it's yogurt, not cream or sour cream in everything—crab cakes, risotto, even cheesecake!

Greek yogurt is such a fantastic hunger killer that it can help you lose a lot of weight in just a little time. Years ago, when I was bloated, overweight, and unhappy, Dr. Nikolaides shared with me his secret, an easy way to drop nearly ten pounds in two weeks. What you do is eat a bowl of yogurt and drink a cup of Greek mountain tea, a traditional herbal blend in Greece, every night for dinner for two weeks, while eating what you normally would for breakfast and lunch (but remember, *metron ariston,* "everything in moderation"). The combination of cold yogurt and hot tea for dinner fills you up wonderfully—I was amazed at how satisfied and fulfilled I felt on this simple meal. When I tried it, I lost nearly ten pounds in two weeks without even trying and not once feeling hungry! I would go to bed happy and full; the following morning, I would walk out of the house feeling lighter and thinner. To try it for yourself, see our complete Kick-Start Yogurt Plan on page 29! (Note: Weight loss on the Kick-Start Yogurt Plan will vary by individual. For this plan and any other weight-loss diet, please consult with your doctor before you start.)

GROWING UP ON GREEK YOGURT

My grandmother used to say yogurt was the food for everyone in the family, from our little babies to the very, very old—it's so gentle on your body and easy to eat that everybody can have it! Growing up, we always had a big bowl of homemade yogurt in our kitchen, and we ate from it every day. When my siblings and I complained to our parents about being hungry, they didn't have junk food to give us like a lot of parents feed kids today (potato chips, cookies, and the other packaged "foods")—they told us to go eat yogurt!

But the yogurt my family had was much different from the yogurt most people eat today, even the packaged Greek yogurt that's become so popular. In Greece, it was not the custom to buy yogurt—we always made it! Our yogurt was fresher, creamier, thicker, richer, and tangier than any you can imagine—unless you've been to my restaurants, where we make yogurt using my mother's recipe. She was the one in our family who led the yogurt-making, and I was the only child who would stay by her side to watch, learn, and help. She started by heating the milk on the stove in a giant pot, sticking her finger in it to make sure it was just the perfect temperature. Since you need yogurt to make yogurt, she would add to the pot a cup from the last batch we had in the house. Once the ingredients in the pot were ready, I would tell my sisters to bring me their blankets and help me cover the pot—it was so much fun for us to "put the yogurt to bed," it became a family ritual! In several hours, it would thicken into a heavy, creamy paste. We would bundle up this tangy paste in cheesecloth and hang it from a rope in the kitchen so it could drain and become even thicker. This would take hours, sometimes going through the night, but I would get so impatient waiting for the yogurt to drain that I would ask one of my sisters to help me take the bundle down so I could taste it. And oh, the flavor! So tart, but still creamy and refreshing. My mouth waters now just thinking about it. You can taste it yourself by following my mother's prized homemade yogurt recipe on page 268.

Like many Mediterranean families, we always got together for a big afternoon meal on Sundays, but our meal was made up mostly of yogurt. My grandmother cooked the Sunday dinner, using yogurt to tenderize the meat (the one time per week we ate meat) and to make a sauce to serve the meat with, whether it was chicken or lamb. Our pasta and rice dishes were made creamy with yogurt, and there was always a big bowl of homemade yogurt on the table in case we wanted to add some to any dish—and I always did!

Our family also ate a lot of tzatziki, a traditional Greek yogurt sauce made with cucumbers, olive oil, lemon juice, herbs, and a touch of vinegar. My grandmother would serve it with bread, meat, vegetables, and salad—one of the best sauces in the world! In Greece, they say that if you want your food to taste better, you eat tzatziki because the combination of yogurt and cucumber opens up your palate and enhances the flavor of food.

As children, we loved yogurt so much that it was our food of choice when we had food fights. My sisters and I would scoop it up like snow and throw it in each other's faces. And it was good for us! I would rub the yogurt all over my face and body because I knew from my grandmother it helps hydrate your skin, making it soft and smooth. She would use yogurt as a beauty mask when all the men were out in the field, saying it was better—and better for you—than any other beauty remedy. She also mixed yogurt with egg yolks to use as a sunscreen and as a salve for the burns I would get in the kitchen and over the fire as a young chef.

My Grandmother's Yogurt Mask

WHAT WE NEED

1 cup 2% plain Greek yogurt

1 teaspoon grated lemon zest

WHAT WE DO

Mix the yogurt and lemon zest together in a small bowl. Coat your face with the yogurt mixture—you can even use this gentle mask on the sensitive skin around your eyes. Leave the mask on for 1 hour. Rinse off with warm water. Feel refreshed and have softer, smoother, healthier skin!

THE YOGURT EXPERIENCE TODAY

Greek yogurt is the second most important ingredient I use in my kitchen, following olive oil. We make our own yogurt using organic 2% milk, because the added fat makes it creamier and more filling than yogurt containing less fat. (For more on the benefits of 2% yogurt, see "Full-Fat vs. Fat-Free vs. 2%" on page 72.) We use yogurt in so many of our dishes, it's almost impossible to count them. Here are some examples:

- Sauces for pasta, rice, fish, and meat
- Soups
- Marinades for chicken, lamb, and beef
- Dips like hummus, spinach dip, and, of course, tzatziki!
- Dressings for salads, potatoes, and vegetables
- Desserts like cheesecake, ice cream, pie, and custard
- Baked goods
- As a garnish on plates

Greek yogurt gives food the perfect blend of flavors because it's creamy and rich, yet tart at the same time. Like butter and cream, Greek yogurt gives food a lush, rich feeling in your mouth, but to me, the taste of yogurt is purer, better—and it's much lower in calories and higher in protein and other healthy nutrients.

I use yogurt in recipes where other chefs use milk, cream, mayonnaise, or sour cream. For example, I don't add butter or milk to mashed potatoes, I add Greek yogurt—this turns the normally fattening side into a rich, high-protein dish. And one of my favorite yogurt creations is Hortosoupa (page 185), a green pea soup made from only fresh green peas, leeks, olive oil, onion, and yogurt—you can taste every single ingredient, giving the soup a wonderful earthiness.

You don't need to do much to Greek yogurt to turn it into a sensual dessert—just add honey and it's a healthy, tasty treat all on its own! At my restaurants, we serve very simple yogurt parfaits, layered with fruit and honey in beautifully curved, clear glasses. We also use Greek yogurt to make cheesecake, custard, flan, and, my favorite, ice cream! You can do this at home by putting Greek yogurt into an ice cream maker with honey and fresh fruit. The taste is creamier and tangier than regular ice cream, but lighter and not heavy and bloating like ice cream. The honey adds antioxidants and makes the ice cream taste naturally sweet, not sugary. Sometimes, I even add baklava for a very sweet—and very Greek!—yogurt treat. But my favorite flavor of frozen Greek yogurt is made with blueberries. It's so rich and smooth, and you can taste the beautiful flavor of the berries. (See page 263 for the recipe.)

We also bake using yogurt in place of butter in cakes, cookies, brownies, pie crusts, and quick breads. Yogurt keeps these baked goods tasting moist and is much richer and more flavorful than applesauce, which some home chefs use as a fat substitute. I also use yogurt to make homemade frosting. You can concoct any flavor by mixing yogurt with a little honey, then adding chocolate, vanilla, or fresh fruit.

I gave away to the entire world my secret recipe using Greek yogurt when I was on *Good Morning, America*. If you want to taste the most flavorful, moistest spanakopita (the very famous Greek spinach pie) you've ever had, don't make it with just cheese—use yogurt! This makes it creamy, fluffy, and slightly tart, balancing the savory flavor of the phyllo dough for perfect harmony. I shared this secret with the chefs at the White House when I cooked for President Obama and his guests, and they absolutely loved it! (See page 206 for the recipe.)

THE YOGURT CLEANSE

Greek yogurt isn't just for losing weight—this superfood also cleans out all the toxins in your body. Yogurt is one of the best natural sources of healthy probiotics, which counter all the bad bacteria and build-up in your body. But unlike juice cleanses and other quick-fix diets, yogurt gives your body protein, calcium, and other minerals you need to stay strong while your body flushes out the bad stuff. Whenever I go on my yogurt cleanse, I feel like a new person afterward—I feel like singing! You should also have a lot of yogurt whenever you are sick, whether you have a cold, the flu, or a digestive illness. All of yogurt's good bacteria will help boost your immune system and make your bowels move properly if you are constipated or have diarrhea.

PILLAR TWO

Greek Yogurt (Science)

O VER THE LAST DECADE, Greek yogurt has gone from relative obscurity in the United States to become one of the trendiest, most popular foods on store shelves today. Take a trip to the yogurt section in the dairy aisle of almost any supermarket, and you'll see primarily Greek yogurt brands and blends. Walk around a little more, and you'll find Greek yogurt added to all sorts of packaged creations, from salad dressing and ice cream to hummus, granola bars, and cereal. There is a good reason for Greek yogurt's epidemic popularity: Not only does it taste good, it's good for your body—and your body's ability to burn fat. Here are three reasons Greek yogurt needs to be in your fat-burning arsenal:

1. GREEK YOGURT IS HIGHER IN FAT-BURNING PROTEIN THAN ALMOST ANY OTHER FOOD.

Greek yogurt contains significantly more hunger-stopping protein per ounce than almost any other ready-to-eat food. One cup contains 23 grams of protein—more than double the amount found in the same-size serving of low-fat fruit yogurt (10 grams). Here's how Greek yogurt stacks up:

FOOD	PROTEIN (GRAMS)	CALORIES
2% plain Greek yogurt, 8 oz.	23	170
Low-fat fruit yogurt, 8 oz.	10	245
Almonds, 1 oz.	8	165
Beans, 4 oz.	8	130
Cheddar cheese, 1 oz.	7	115
Egg, large	6	75
Chicken breast, cooked, 3 oz.	24	165

Why care about protein? Research shows eating high-protein foods like Greek yogurt curbs hunger, increases satiety (the feeling of fullness), stabilizes blood-sugar levels, reduces cravings, and prevents overeating. What's more, your body burns more calories metabolizing and digesting protein than it does carbohydrates. Known as the thermal effect of food, this pleasant benefit of eating protein can make a big difference on your daily energy intake by slashing the calorie count of the foods you eat by as much as 30 percent. For example, if you consume a 100-calorie cup of high-protein Greek yogurt, your body only ingests 70 to 80 percent of those calories, or 70 to 80 calories total. Lastly, eating a high-protein diet helps promote and preserve muscle tone, helping you drop fat, not muscle, when losing weight. This isn't important only for aesthetic reasons, but also to aid in further weight loss, since muscle burns significantly more calories than body fat does, even while at rest.

As an added bonus, Greek yogurt also has fewer carbs, less sugar, and less sodium than regular yogurt. A cup of 2% plain Greek yogurt has 9 grams of carbs, 9 grams of sugar, and about 75 milligrams of sodium. The same-size serving of low-fat plain yogurt clocks in with 17 grams of carbs, 17 grams of sugar, and 171 milligrams of sodium! Here's how the two stack up:

1 CUP OF 2% PLAIN GREEK YOGURT	
Calories	170
Calories from fat	40
Total fat	4.5 g
Saturated fat	3 g
Trans fat	0
Cholesterol	15 mg
Sodium	75 mg
Total carbohydrates	9 g
Fiber	0 g
Sugars	9 g
Protein	23 g

1 CUP OF LOW-FAT PLAIN YOGURT	
Calories	155
Calories from fat	33
Total fat	4 g
Saturated fat	2 g
Trans fat	0
Cholesterol	15 mg
Sodium	171 mg
Total carbohydrates	17 g
Fiber	0 g
Sugars	17 g
Protein	13 g

2. GREEK YOGURT IS ONE OF THE FEW FOODS TO CONTAIN THE GOOD-FOR-YOU BACTERIA YOUR BODY NEEDS TO PROMOTE DIGESTION AND LOSE WEIGHT.

Protein isn't Greek yogurt's only important feature. For one thing, other foods, mainly meats, are also high in protein. But Greek yogurt has another remarkable benefit. It is chock-full of something almost no other common food contains: probiotics. This good-for-you bacteria has become a very hot topic in the health world of late, and for good reason: Reams of research continue to credit these tiny organisms with fighting colds, curing diarrhea, preventing allergies, boosting the immune system, and even combating cancer and heart disease. But now, new research shows probiotics may be the *key* to permanent weight loss. Let's take a look.

Did you know you have ten times more bacteria in your body than you have cells? Most of us never stop to think about it, but there's a tiny ecosystem of millions of microorganisms living in our guts, driving basic functions like digestion and influencing our overall health every day. This community of so-called microbiota is made up of both beneficial bacteria like probiotics and some not-so-friendly microbes that can make us sick. And just like the environment we live in, if we get too much of one kind of bacteria, even a healthy germ, it can throw our whole gastrointestinal ecology out of whack, slowing down the metabolism and inhibiting the body's ability to burn fat.

Scientists first got a glimpse of the crucial role bacteria play in weight loss almost a decade ago, when a breakthrough study published in the journal *Nature* showed that overweight people have different microbiotas than lean people. Since then, a number of studies have reached similar conclusions, including a revolutionary 2013 experiment in Japan showing the most successful weight-loss operation, gastric bypass surgery, causes such significant fat loss simply because the surgery readjusts the microbe levels in patients' bodies. The message is becoming the same: If you don't have the right kind of germs in your body, you'll have a hard time losing weight, no matter how little you eat or how much you exercise.

So how common is it to have a bacterial imbalance? Extremely. In fact, it's so common in most Western countries that one American doctor wrote in the *Huffington Post* that she can count on two hands how many patients she's seen with the right amount of gut germs. The reason for this is that many modern foods, drugs, and lifestyle habits affect our gut flora. Taking antibiotics, antacids, over-the-counter pain medications, laxatives, or antidiarrheal drugs will throw your gut ecology out of balance. Exposure to certain pollutants and pesticides in food, water, and the environment can create unhealthy microbe levels. You'll also disrupt your gut flora if you don't drink enough water every day, or if you consume artificial sweeteners like Splenda and Equal. Finally, eating according to the Standard American Diet (SAD)—high in sugar and unhealthy fat—is one of the best ways to kick your gut ecology into disarray. One study even found that when mice were fed to match the SAD for just one day, the microbe levels in their bodies drastically changed.

If it's so easy to throw your gut bacteria out of whack, what can you do to change your microbiota—and actually lose weight instead of gaining it? Eat more yogurt. When consumed, this food containing live cultures is the easiest, most pleasurable way to get the daily dose of probiotics your body needs to bring your microbiota back into a fat-burning zone. Sure, there are other foods that contain probiotics, including raw sauerkraut, tempeh, miso, and the fermented tea kombucha, but it's difficult (and costly) to eat enough tempeh or drink enough kombucha on a daily basis to right a gastrointestinal imbalance. What's more, if you make your own yogurt using Maria's famous recipe (page 268), you'll double your probiotic intake, since homemade yogurt has significantly more probiotics than packaged products do. Finally, if you think you can take a probiotic supplement to balance your gut flora, think again: Studies show our bodies absorb nutrients through food far better than in compressed pills or potions.

FULL-FAT vs. FAT-FREE vs. 2%

We like 2%—and science does, too. For just 4 calories more per ounce than the fat-free variety, Greek yogurt with 2% fat is also creamier, richer, more filling, and more satisfying, meaning you'll eat less overall and not be as tempted to eat again for hours afterward. Studies also show that when you eat any carbohydrate-containing food with fat, like 2% yogurt, the fat works to slow your body's blood sugar response to carbohydrate, causing your body to release less of the fat-storing hormone insulin. In other words, 2% Greek yogurt is lower on the glycemic index than fat-free yogurt. Finally, *Consumer Reports* found people overwhelmingly preferred the taste of 2% over fat-free. In short, 2% Greek yogurt is a true pleasure food, one you'll want to eat and enjoy eating, making it central to the Greek Diet.

So what about full-fat Greek yogurt? This option has 11 calories more per ounce than fat-free, but it also has a whopping 7 grams of saturated fat. While doctors now believe some saturated fat in moderation is beneficial to heart health (contradicting an outdated mandate that any type of saturated fat was bad), the jury is still out on how much saturated fat is too much.

3. THE CALCIUM IN GREEK YOGURT HELPS STIMULATE WEIGHT LOSS BETTER THAN OTHER FOODS.

Calcium isn't just good for your bones. Numerous studies have found that eating dairy foods high in calcium, like yogurt, helps increase your ability to break down fat while maintaining your metabolism, which drops when you lose weight. But you can't just pop a calcium supplement and expect to see results: Research shows consuming calcium and protein together is the magic bullet for weight loss—one without the other won't necessarily do the trick. Greek yogurt, with 250 milligrams of calcium and 23 grams of protein per cup, has one of the highest ratios of both fat-fighting nutrients naturally found in almost any food.

Studies also suggest there may just be something special about eating yogurt in itself that stimulates weight loss. A study from the University of Tennessee at Knoxville found that people who ate 18 ounces of high-calcium, high-protein yogurt a day (that's over 2 cups) lost 22 percent more weight and 61 percent more body fat than those who didn't indulge in the creamy food. The yogurt eaters in the study also maintained one-third more calorie-burning muscle mass while losing weight than the people who didn't eat yogurt, helping the yogurt eaters stay toned and lean.

PILLAR THREE
Vegetables (Sensual)

WHEN I CAME TO NEW YORK and opened my restaurant, a lot of people told me New Yorkers were picky eaters. I didn't believe them. I thought to myself, how could people living in the culinary center of the world not be adventurous? So I created my menu as I wanted, with lots of vegetable, bean, and seafood dishes, and gauged the reaction during my opening.

What I discovered was that New Yorkers were not picky eaters—they were healthy eaters! Many people were vegetarians, too, but they were afraid to wear their dietary choice on their sleeve for fear of being mocked or scolded. But no Greek chef would mock a vegetarian—our food is teaming with vegetables, often served as the main attraction of a meal, not hidden behind a meat entrée. Yet I found my vegetable dishes were also tempting to omnivores, even carnivores. This helped solidify my presence in the city and allowed me to befriend my customers and expose them to new and exciting dishes—what more could a chef want?

Vegetables are essential to the Greek diet, both in ancient times and modern days. Greece's warm and wet climate has made the country lush with vegetation, a rich breeding ground for the growth of all kinds of vegetables. Wild greens cover the mountains and valleys and make up a large part of the diet. As seasonal eaters, the people of Greece embody the new trendy American ideal of eating seasonal and local cuisine. But in Greece, this is not a new concept, but an ancient one.

VEGETABLES IN ANCIENT GREECE

The ancient Greeks relied heavily on vegetables to add variety to their diet and had access to a plethora of wild greens, asparagus, beets, radishes, onions, and garlic. They would cook these vegetables in soups or eat them raw, along with cooked beans and whole grains such as wheat and barley.

Traditional Greek cuisine has a strong association with many vegetables, including tomatoes, corn, and potatoes, but some of these didn't exist in ancient Greece, and were introduced to Europe from America. Spinach, now a Greek staple, didn't come to Greece from Asia until the Middle Ages.

Still, vegetables were imperative to the Greek diet in ancient times, as they are today. One of the most famous Greek mathematicians of all time, Pythagoras, was also one of the earliest advocates of vegetarianism. He believed in metempsychosis, the transmigration of souls into the bodies of other animals, and thought it was unhealthy and sacrilegious to consume animal protein.

GROWING UP A FARMER'S DAUGHTER

As a child, my mother would insist that my siblings and I drink vegetable broth twice a week. She would save all the scraps, roots, and tips of vegetables we didn't use in cooking and make the broth by boiling them in a big pot on the stove. When I asked her why we had to drink the broth so often, she told me that it was giving us all the necessary vitamins, minerals, and nutrients that we might otherwise have lost by not eating every part of our vegetables. This, in turn, would keep us healthy all year long. To flavor the broth, she would grind stalks of celery into a paste using a mortar and pestle. Celery has a salty taste, so adds a briny flavor to food without any added sodium. To this day, I still add celery to my dishes to try to cut down on the salt I use when cooking.

When I was a young girl, I cried for a whole week after I stepped on a cucumber vine. When my grandmother asked me why I was crying, I told her I had ruined the cucumbers. But she said it was a good thing I destroyed the *aguri,* or cucumber, because now we could make a medicine to help clear my sinuses. She made a juice out of the crushed cucumbers and gave it to me to use to wash out my sinuses, like many people do with a neti pot. The cucumber juice stung, but I didn't have a sinus problem for the rest of the year.

Some of my favorite snacks as a child were made from vegetables. I made my own version of tzatziki, or Greek yogurt sauce, by slicing a cucumber, putting a dollop of my mother's yogurt on top, and finishing it with a slice of garlic—delicious! (For my tzatziki recipe now, see page 271.) I would also take leaves of the wild purslane growing in our backyard and wrap them in larger kale or arugula leaves with feta (and sometimes tomato) to make my own creation. Years later, this "recipe" inspired me to create vegetarian Greek sushi, a popular appetizer among my patrons.

How to Use Celery Instead of Salt

In any recipe that calls for salt, you can use celery to replace some of the sodium. The trick works best for high-heat cooking methods, like grilling, sautéing, stewing, and braising, but also flavors foods nicely in a slow cooker! Finely dice a stalk or two of celery and add to your pot, pan, or slow cooker. One diced celery stalk can take the place of about ½ teaspoon salt.

VEGETABLES TODAY

Nowadays, after importing many of the Americanized dietary habits, Greeks eat far fewer vegetables than they used to several decades ago. The result has been an epidemic of expanding waistlines and worsening health. Recently, many Greeks have tried to counter these effects by going back to the old ways of eating.

For years, eating lots of vegetables was part of the traditional Greek diet, including wild greens like kale, spinach, Swiss chard, dandelion greens, mustard greens, beet greens, chicory, and purslane; mushrooms, zucchini, summer squash, onions, leeks, fennel, eggplant, beets, cauliflower, asparagus, peppers, cabbage, green beans, celery, carrots, potatoes, pumpkin, winter squash, peas, cucumbers, artichokes, lettuce, and radishes. Since ancient times, vegetables not native to Greece have been introduced and incorporated into the cuisine, and adopted as its own.

The majority of the Greek Diet is made up of vegetables, prepared in any way you want, whether grilled, sautéed, braised, boiled, roasted, steamed, or raw. We encourage you to recombine the same basic ingredients with different cooking methods and create new and interesting dishes, just as traditional Greeks do. For example, rethink basic boiled green beans by sautéing them with tomatoes and a touch of olive oil, salt, pepper, and oregano—an easy side dish for a delicately grilled piece of fish. Or slow-cook the same ingredients in an oven at 350°F for an hour or so to turn them into a hearty stew, perfect for a main dish. The addition of herbs and spices makes this dish even healthier, but we'll get to that in a later pillar (Pillar Eight: Herbs and Spices).

COOKING WITH VEGETABLES

At my restaurants, vegetables and vegetarian dishes make up a large portion of my menu. I take great pride in teaching my kitchen staff the proper way to prepare dishes in the Greek style. A lot of the Greek cooking methods are quite simple, like grilling and roasting, but require time and care in order to maintain the flavor, freshness, and integrity of the vegetables themselves. In my kitchens and on the Greek Diet, we don't add unnecessary fat to make vegetables taste better, or hide them in heavy sauces. Instead, if you learn to highlight their natural flavor and let them shine, you'll be rewarded with a tastier—and healthier—dish.

For example, I make a dish called *kounoupidi,* or cauliflower, that is easy, and inexpensive for any home chef to make. I braise the cauliflower florets in fresh marinara sauce (you can opt for store-bought sauce made without sugar) instead of boiling them in water or frying them. This way, you don't lose the vitamins or nutrients, and it doesn't get mushy. Patrons love this dish and tell me how flavorful it is—you will too if you try it at home (see page 201)!

One of the most well-known Greek dishes is spanakopita, or spinach pie. But I prefer a similar dish called *hortopita,* which literally translates to "wild greens pie." Instead of using only spinach in the pie, I add Swiss chard and kale, along with different onion varieties like shallots and scallions, and many herbs to help balance the flavor. The result is a pie that's moist but not soggy, flavorful but not overwhelming, and healthy because it includes many different leafy greens and nutrients. For my hortopita recipe, see page 208.

How to Blanch Vegetables

Blanching is a cooking technique usually reserved for vegetables and fruits that helps maintain the texture and nutrients of a food. To blanch a fruit or vegetable, quickly plunge it in boiling water, then remove it and submerge it in ice water to stop the cooking process. Total blanching time varies by the item you're blanching and how well you want it cooked.

PILLAR THREE
Vegetables (Science)

YOU KNOW VEGETABLES ARE GOOD FOR YOU, but do you know they are imperative to losing weight—and keeping that weight off? In today's age of diet crazes that include everything from eating only protein to consuming only shakes, many of us seem to have forgotten that eating vegetables themselves—the original plant food—is the best and easiest way to lose weight. Here's why.

1. THE MORE VEGETABLES YOU EAT, THE FEWER CALORIES YOU CONSUME, THE MORE WEIGHT YOU LOSE.

Think of vegetables as your "free food." Most vegetables, with the exception of starchy white and sweet potatoes, corn, and winter squash, are so low in calories, you can eat as much as you want and still lose weight. Having a free food is extremely helpful to hungry dieters—you always have something to snack on!

Interestingly, studies also show we tend to eat the same weight in food every day. So if you can simply switch some of the fattening weight you eat—red meat, processed grains and breads, and packaged snack foods—to vegetables, you can still eat the same amount of food while taking in a lot fewer calories.

Americans love their superlatives: the safest car to buy, the funniest television show to watch, the best place to live. But with vegetables, the best ones are those you'll eat the most often. So if you like asparagus and tomatoes, go crazy. Or if peppers and onions are your preference, do it. Just keep in mind that the wider the range of vegetables you eat is, the wider your exposure to a range of micronutrients that play important roles in your metabolism and fat-burning abilities.

The only caveat: Be mindful of your intake of starchy vegetables, primarily white and sweet potatoes, peas, corn, pumpkin, and winter squash. These vegetables are higher in carbohydrates, or sugar, often lower in water and fiber, and more calorically dense than nonstarchy vegetables. *But* starchy vegetables, even white potatoes, are a far smarter choice for weight loss than are most foods, including meat, cheese, and processed grains like pasta, bagels, cereal, and crackers. They are lower in calories and higher in fiber, water, and micronutrients than 99.9 percent of foods in the Standard American Diet. Starchy vegetables, particularly potatoes, also contain a type of fiber called resistant starch. This starch creates fatty acids in the large intestine that help block the body's ability to absorb carbohydrates.

2. VEGETABLES HAVE MORE MICRONUTRIENTS PER CALORIE THAN ANY OTHER FOOD, REVVING METABOLISM AND FEEDING YOUR BODY THE NUTRIENTS IT NEEDS TO LOSE WEIGHT.

It's a fact: Calorie for calorie, vegetables contain more fat-fighting micronutrients—vitamins, minerals, antioxidants, and phytochemicals—than any other food. Why does that matter for weight loss? Well, if you're deficient, or even moderately low, in micronutrients, you won't have enough energy, your metabolism won't function properly, and you will *not* lose weight.

The main reason micronutrients are key to weight loss is that they ensure every system in your body is working properly, from your circulatory system (including your heart) and your digestive system to your metabolism. For example, if you're not getting enough B vitamins, magnesium, and other nutrients, your metabolism can slow to such a crawl that no matter how little you eat, your body won't be able to burn fat to lose weight.

Micronutrients like vitamins, minerals, and antioxidants are also essential to boosting energy. These nutrients work synergistically to fuel your body with the energy it needs to move more, exercise, and take the stairs instead of the elevator. Having more energy also allows you to make smart food choices: Research suggests that when we're fatigued, we're more likely to give in to junk food, which in turn only saps our energy more.

Finally, micronutrients, especially antioxidants, are necessary to combat cell-damaging free radicals and help remove waste from cells. Allow yourself to become overrun with free radicals and other cellular waste, and you'll create a state of chronic inflammation in your body. This will thwart even the best efforts to lose weight: Like an inflamed knee or hip, an inflamed body can't move well or function properly, causing your natural fat-burning abilities to flag while your body focuses on trying to lower inflammation and heal.

Substituting Supplements for Kale and Broccoli

If you think you can pop a multivitamin instead of eating vegetables and foods to get all the nutrients you need to lose weight, think again: Studies show our bodies don't absorb nutrients from supplements and fortified foods (foods with nutrients artificially added) nearly as well as they do from foods that naturally contain these nutrients.

---

3. VEGETABLES KILL HUNGER WITH THEIR UNIQUE DOUBLE WHAMMY OF WATER AND FIBER.

Most Americans don't think of vegetables as hunger-fighting food—but that's just one reason we're fat and quickly getting fatter. Stop looking to processed junk like granola bars and potato chips to satiate your stomach and start considering Mother Nature's best bounty: veggies! Vegetables curb hunger pangs better than most foods because they wield a rare double whammy: They contain high amounts of both water and fiber.

Your body is made up of 60 to 70 percent water, and every part of you, including your brain, hormones, metabolism, and stomach, depends on adequate water intake to function properly. Don't consume enough water and your thinking will be foggy, your hormones will be out of whack, your digestion will malfunction, your metabolism will slow, and your body won't be able to burn fat.

Out of all foods, vegetables and fruits have the highest water content, with vegetables averaging around 90 percent water. Vegetables' high water content triggers weight loss in three ways. First, it helps prevent even the mildest form of dehydration that can thwart your metabolism and body's fat-burning ability. Second, water increases the volume of a food without adding calories. The more volume to a food, the more it fills you up and keeps you feeling full for longer.

Water's filling effect is even more pronounced when combined with fiber—a relative rarity among foods. In fact, vegetables and fruits are the only two foods groups with both a high water and fiber content. Many vegetables are packed with soluble fiber, a type of fiber that works with water to form a gel that expands in your stomach to make you feel full, even uncomfortably at times (you'll recognize this feeling if you've ever eaten too much broccoli or too many Brussels sprouts). The feeling of satiety from soluble fiber is so effective that companies bottle the fiber in weight-loss drugs that don't work as well—nor are they as safe!—as a simple spinach salad or several cups of crispy, delicious kale chips. Finally, vegetables also contain insoluble fiber, which adds bulk to foods and works like a natural laxative, helping speed the digestive process. For more details on how fiber speeds weight loss, see Pillar Four: Beans.

To conceptualize just how filling the double whammy of water and fiber is, which one of the following would make you feel fuller:

- Five cups of broccoli OR half of one Twinkie? (150 calories)
- Two and a half cups of green beans OR one ounce of cheddar cheese? (100 calories)
- Three cups of cooked kale OR eleven potato chips? (100 calories)
- One small baked sweet potato or a half tablespoon of butter? (55 calories)

All of these choices have the same number of calories. But it's obvious which will fill you up more and leave you feeling full longer.

FOUR FAST WAYS TO EAT MORE VEGETABLES

1. Snack on fresh veggies whenever you're hungry: baby carrots, celery, sliced bell peppers (red, orange, and green), steamed or raw broccoli, cherry tomatoes, cucumbers, even roasted eggplant or steamed asparagus spears.
2. Make vegetables the main feature of every meal: Spinach or kale with eggs or in a shake for breakfast, a big salad for lunch, butternut squash pasta for dinner. Use Maria's creative ways or find your own style of making vegetables the primary component of your meals.
3. Have a bowl of broth-based vegetable soup before dinner. Studies show the combo of hot water and veggies helps fill you up and prevents overeating during meals. ·
4. When ordering out, ask to substitute starchy sides like potatoes, French fries, and rice with a salad or grilled or steamed vegetables.

INSTEAD OF:	Calories	HAVE THIS:	Calories
Rice, 1 cup cooked	205	Spinach, 1 cup	7
Ground beef (80% lean), 3 oz. cooked	230	Grilled mushrooms, 3 oz.	40
Potato chips, 1 cup	150	Baked kale chips, 1 cup	20
Wheat Thins, 8 small	80	Baby carrots, 8 large	30
Regular pancake, 1 large	200	Zucchini pancake, 1 large	60
Mashed potatoes, 1 cup	240	Mashed cauliflower, 1 cup	50
Alfredo sauce, ½ cup	220	Tomato sauce, ½ cup	50
French fries, 1 small order	200	Artichoke, 1 steamed	60
Guacamole, 1 cup	450	Mashed peas with yogurt, 1 cup	150
Spaghetti, 1 cup cooked	220	Spaghetti squash, 1 cup cooked	40

Raw vs. Cooked?

Despite what some raw-foods zealots say, cooked vegetables are just as good for speeding weight loss as raw vegetables are. Cooking vegetables breaks down cell walls, making micronutrients more absorbable and digestible. However, cooking vegetables for long durations at high temperatures or in large amounts of water can drain a vegetable's micronutrient contents. Steaming and pan-frying veggies preserve the most micronutrients.

PILLAR FOUR
Beans (Sensual)

WHEN I WAS GROWING UP, I would hear many great things about the *fava* from Santorini, a small Greek island in the Aegean Sea. Fava is a traditional Greek dish made from
pureed split yellow peas (different from actual fava beans or broad beans). I thought to myself,
how could their fava be so special when ours was already delicious? Since we grew our own fava
on our farm, we made it all the time, adding olive oil and lemon for a simple, silky dish.

When I was 28, I finally made it to Santorini for a few hours for a business meeting. My
friend Nikos happened to be there that same day and invited me to join him for lunch. We went
to a taverna in a beautiful village called Oea, and I knew I had to try the fava—I was in Santorini, after all! I ordered the dish and discovered a complicated mixture of peas with chopped
onions, capers, and *ladolemono,* or olive oil lemon sauce. Before I even stuck a spoon in it, I said
to Nikos, "Oh, that's why they say it's the best, because of all the condiments they put on top!"
He told me to just taste it, but I asked, "How can I taste it? Fava is fava. This has so many things."
He knew what I meant and asked for a small plate of plain fava, so I could really see what the
dish was like.

As soon as I tasted the plain fava, I knew why people had talked about the dish for years:
The peas were so flavorful, with a different taste and color from the beans we raised on my family's farm. My mouth was so excited—my taste buds were dancing! And I knew why. Santorini,
originally part of a volcano chain, has a rich, fertile soil, full of minerals and nutrients. The result
was a truly better fava! I didn't even want to try it with the condiments, it was so flavorful and
cooked to perfection. (For a traditional fava recipe, see page 219.)

GROWING UP ON BEANS

On my family's farm, we grew many different types of legumes, including beans and peas. We would harvest them during the summer and let them dry in the sun, so we would have dried beans year-round. In the winter months, we'd use the sun-dried beans in stews, sauces, and casseroles. When the beans were fresh, though, we'd eat them right off the pole that the farmers use to grow the beans. I always thought it was magical to grow a food you could eat year-round in so many different forms.

When I was growing up, some years we had a terrible olive oil shortage in our village. Sometimes there was enough for my family to use, but not enough to sell. Other times, there was not even enough for us to use, so we would have to buy olive oil at cost because we couldn't live without it! During those years, money was tight, and there were many things my family could not afford, especially luxury items like fish and chicken. We went months without any animal protein, but we never suffered—in fact, we grew stronger and healthier every season, consuming mostly beans and *horta* (wild greens).

Some people think beans are boring, but they never knew my grandmother, who would attempt to reinvent the wheel by making all kinds of new dishes out of the same basic ingredients— bean patties, beans with tomato sauce, beans with vinegar, beans with other vegetables, beans with cooked rice or farro (a crunchy, nutty variety of wheat). We even ate beans with cinnamon and honey in a morning stew, similar to oatmeal! For Christmas, she would cook black-eyed peas with pork fat, which was an incredibly tasty treat for my whole family. All year long I would ask her to make them this way, but she would tell me it was only for special occasions, because the animal fat would make my grandfather's cholesterol rise. Whenever I complained about eating so many beans, she would tell me stories about the ancient Greeks and how many beans they ate, which is what helped make them all so beautiful, clever, and thin.

BEANS IN ANCIENT GREECE

When I did the research for the official cookbook I wrote for the Athens 2004 Olympic Games (*Ancient Dining,* ISP International Athletic Editions, 2004), I discovered my grandmother was right about the ancient Greeks: They practically lived on beans and legumes! In ancient times, beans were just as bountiful, inexpensive, and healthful as they are today.

Of all the varieties available today, lentils, chickpeas, peas, and broad beans (called fava beans in the United States) were the most common in ancient Greece. Beans, often called the "poor man's meat," were a main source of protein for the majority of the population, in addition to providing fiber and many important vitamins and antioxidants.

Beans were used not only for food, but in religious and political practices, too. There were many superstitions surrounding beans. For example, the Greeks associated black spots on fava beans with death, and forbade priests to eat them. Beans were also used in the world's first democracy as a voting method: Voting with a white bean was considered a "yes," while black beans were considered a "no." The phrase "the beans have been counted" (*koukia metrimena*) is still used today to refer to election results.

CANNED vs. DRIED BEANS?

I use mostly dried beans because the quality is generally better, and I'm able to sift out any unhealthy-looking beans from the batch. But I don't turn my nose up at canned beans—a great, easy, inexpensive, and convenient way for home chefs and anyone on the Greek Diet to add more beans to meals and salads. Just a few things to keep in mind when cooking with canned beans:

- Rinse canned beans in water before adding to a dish to reduce salt content.
- Add canned beans later in the cooking process to recipes that call for dried beans.
- While most canned beans are fine, opt for using dried lentils; canned lentils often cook too quickly and easily disintegrate.

THE SLIMMING POWER OF BEANS

Beans count for a large portion of my everyday diet—a habit I adopted after gaining so much weight eating a Western diet. During my career as a lobbyist, I usually spent no more than a night or two in any one place, and when I dined out, there were many carbohydrate options on the menus, but few involved beans. Instead, I ate refined pasta and rice dishes and gained nearly forty pounds in ten years! As time passed and my weight continued to increase, I thought back to the stories my grandmother used to tell me about the ancient Greeks being so beautiful, clever, and thin, and decided to make it a point to add beans back to my diet.

As soon as I did, I instantly noticed a change: I felt fuller after meals and throughout the day, my cravings for refined carbs ended, and I began to lose weight. I also started feeling healthier, as though my body was telling me that I was doing the right thing, and it was going to reward me for it.

COOKING WITH BEANS

One of my favorite appetizers is something called Gigantes me Spanaki, or giant beans with tomatoes, herbs, spinach, and olive oil. (For the recipe, see page 218.) During the colder months, I serve a wonderful lentil soup, made delicious by the time spent cooking it, letting it sit for hours on the stove. (You can make my lentil soup easily at home, too, either on the stove or in a slow cooker—see my recipe on page 186.) I also make a cold bean salad with cooked black giant beans, an heirloom variety that adds a unique color and taste, with herbs and a simple red wine vinaigrette. Finally, instead of traditional meatballs and sauce, I make a veggie meatball out of mashed red lentils, herbs, salt, olive oil, and, my secret ingredient, cumin. Even the pickiest meat-eaters love these lentil meatballs, which are lower in calories and fat and higher in fiber and nutrients than any traditional meatball, no matter what cut of meat you use. (For my red lentil faux meatball recipe, see page 221.)

The Secrets to Using Dried Beans

- Whenever possible, soak dried beans overnight, or for at least 6 hours.

- After soaking, skim the floating beans and discard—floating beans generally indicate they were dried past their prime.

- Thoroughly rinse soaked beans before cooking.

- Different varieties of beans call for different cooking methods. Follow the instructions in each recipe carefully to ensure the best taste and texture.

PILLAR FOUR
Beans (Science)

TAKE A MOMENT TO THINK ABOUT the kind of side dishes most Americans eat at home or out at restaurants. Your list likely includes items like mashed potatoes, mac 'n' cheese, rice, spaghetti, and bread. While some of these foods are fine in moderation, most are high in sugar, low in micronutrients like vitamins and minerals, and devoid of the kind of macronutrients that fight fat: fiber, protein, and healthy fat.

The ancient Greeks ate plenty of healthy whole-grain bread, but their starchy side of choice wasn't rice or, worse, manufactured macaroni and cheese out of a box. Instead, they preferred to eat their fish and vegetables with a side of beans. In fact, many Greeks consider their national dish to be a bean-based soup called *fasolada,* made with tomatoes, onions, carrots, celery, and olive oil (see Maria's recipe on page 191). The fact that Greeks consumed copious amounts of beans is a big reason the Mediterranean diet has earned its reputation for lowering heart disease and fighting fat. Here's why:

EAT MORE, WEIGH LESS WITH BEANS

A recent study found that adults who eat lots of beans weigh, on average, 7 pounds fewer than non–bean eaters, even though the bean eaters eat up to 200 calories more per day.

---

1. BEANS HAVE MORE OF THE RIGHT KINDS OF FIBER FOR FAT LOSS THAN ANY OTHER FOOD.

No wonder two-thirds of Americans are fat. Only 3 percent of the country eats enough fiber every day! And that's a huge problem for a number of reasons. Not only does fiber make food more filling, it also slows the release of sugar into the bloodstream. Studies also show a high fiber intake helps lower cholesterol and chronic disease like heart disease, diabetes, and cancer.

But not all fiber is created equal when it comes to weight loss and reaping the macronutrient's many health benefits. Isolate or functional fiber—or fiber that is manufactured in labs and then added to packaged and processed foods like cereal, bread, crackers, supplements, even yogurt—does not seem to have the same health and weight-loss benefits as intact fiber, which is found naturally in food, especially beans. Research shows that a diet high in intact fiber from beans, fruits, vegetables, and whole grains is more effective in making you feel full, lowering your blood sugar, and causing weight loss than a high-fiber diet from isolated fibers.

When it comes to naturally occurring fiber, you need two types to help you lose weight: soluble fiber and insoluble fiber. No other single food has more of both of these types than beans. Here's why you need both:

Soluble fiber dissolves in water. This means that when you eat foods with a lot of soluble fiber, like beans, the nutrient dissolves in liquids in your stomach to form a viscous gel. This gel expands, making you feel fuller longer while holding on to the foods in your stomach longer, an effect known as gastric emptying.

The soluble fiber found in beans also stimulates the release of digestive enzymes that slow the rate at which calories enter our bloodstream. The slower the rate, the less insulin our bodies produce. Insulin is a huge deal when it comes to weight loss: High levels of this hormone in your blood is not only a precursor to diabetes, it also causes our bodies to store fat and interferes with the production of leptin, the "hunger hormone" that tells our brains when we're full.

Insoluble fiber, also found in rich quantities in beans, absorbs water rather than dissolving in it, which also helps us lose weight. When insoluble fiber absorbs water, the fiber adds bulk to the digestive system, working overtime with soluble fiber to make us feel more full.

Insoluble fiber also acts as a natural laxative, speeding the passage of food through the digestive system. This prevents constipation, but also works to clear toxins from our system that can wreak havoc on metabolism and digestion.

Legumes vs. Beans

Botanically speaking, all beans are legumes, a class of plants that also includes lentils, peas, soybeans, and peanuts. For the sake of the Greek Diet, when we talk about beans and their fat-fighting power, we include lentils and soybeans, too, since these legumes are also high in stomach-filling fiber and protein. Peas and peanuts, on the other hand, have nutrient properties more similar to vegetables and nuts, respectively, and you'll find these legumes discussed in more detail in Pillar Three and Pillar Eleven.

Only 3 percent of Americans actually consume the recommended amount of daily fiber: at least 25 grams for women, and at least 38 grams for men.

For optimal weight loss, soluble is the ideal fiber, although you want a balance of both. Look at the following chart showing the foods highest in naturally occurring, or intact, fiber per serving. No food contains more soluble fiber *and* insoluble fiber than beans.

SOLUBLE AND INSOLUBLE FIBER IN FOODS*

FOOD	SERVING SIZE	TOTAL FIBER (G)	SOLUBLE FIBER (G)	INSOLUBLE FIBER (G)
Black beans, cooked	½ cup	5.5	2	3.5
Kidney beans, cooked	½ cup	6.0	3	3
Lima beans, cooked	½ cup	6.5	3.5	3
Navy beans, cooked	½ cup	6	2	4
Northern beans, cooked	½ cup	5.5	5	0.5
Pinto beans, cooked	½ cup	7	2	5
Lentils, cooked	½ cup	8	1	7
All Bran cereal	⅓ cup	8	0.7	7.3
Oatmeal, cooked	½ cup	2	1	1
Oat bran	½ cup	3	2	1
Shredded wheat	⅔ cup	3	0.3	2.7
Wheat germ	⅔ cup	8	1	7
Brussels sprouts, cooked	½ cup	4.5	3.0	1.5
Artichoke, fresh	½ cup	4	3	1
Apple	1 medium	4	1	3

*courtesy NYU Langone Medical Center

2. BEANS CONTAIN FIBER AND PROTEIN, MAKING THEM MORE FILLING THAN MEAT.

Most weight-conscious Americans think of meat, eggs, and potatoes when it comes to filling protein sources, thanks in part to the Atkins diet craze. But these foods don't have anything on beans when it comes to what stops hunger more, since beans have both fiber and protein—the two macronutrients shown to satiate the stomach, keep us fuller longer, and prevent overeating. Better still, beans don't have the hormones, antibiotics, and/or steroids found in commercial meat, or the mercury, PCBs, and other toxins found in seafood.

With the exception of soybeans (and tofu), beans are not a complete protein, meaning they don't have all nine essential amino acids. Specifically, beans lack the essential amino acid lysine—but this protein building block is found in Greek yogurt, nuts, vegetables, and most other Pillar Foods on the Greek Diet.

How much protein do beans have? Some beans, per cup, have as much protein as a serving of meat. Let's compare:

FOOD	PROTEIN (G)
Soybeans, 1 cup	28
Chicken breast, 3 ounces cooked	26
Ground beef (85% lean), 3 ounces cooked	22
Edamame, 1 cup	22
Ham, 3 ounces	19
Lentils, 1 cup cooked	18
Salmon, 3 ounces cooked	17
White beans, 1 cup cooked	17

Beans aren't just good for weight loss. This superfood is also capable of lowering cholesterol and blood pressure while working to prevent heart disease—the number one killer in the United States. A recent study from Arizona State University found that eating ½ cup of beans daily lowered LDL ("bad") cholesterol levels by 8 percent, slashing the risk of heart disease by a whopping 16 percent. Other studies show eating 1 to 2 cups of pinto beans 4 days a week or more can reduce cholesterol by up to an incredible 24 percent. Finally, a third study published in the *Archives of Internal Medicine* found eating 1 cup of beans daily lowers blood pressure, further reducing the risk of heart disease.

Since beans are high in fiber and low on the glycemic index, doctors recommend eating more to ward off type 2 diabetes. A recent study of 64,000 Chinese women found that eating beans and soybeans reduced the risk of type 2 diabetes by 64 percent.

Finally, beans have been shown to prevent and fight off cancer. According to the American Institute of Cancer Research, beans contain natural plant chemicals that inhibit the reproduction of cancerous cells and help slow the growth of tumors. Studies also show that consuming more beans can help prevent breast and colon cancers.

3. BEANS INCLUDE SOME OF THE LOWEST SUGAR CARBOHYDRATES, SATISFYING THE BODY'S NEED FOR CARBS WHILE GIVING US THE ENERGY WE NEED TO BURN FAT.

Have you ever tried to lose weight by not eating any carbs at all? If so, you probably know what it's like to live low-carb, with all the irritability, fatigue, headaches, nausea, weakness, even dizziness associated with the diet. Chances are, you also didn't feel like exercising or even moving much on a low-carb regimen—or when you did, you were not able to go as hard or as long.

Truth is, our bodies need carbs to function well and—surprise—to lose weight. We'll delve more into how carbs help the body burn fat in Pillar Six: Whole Grains, but for now, countless studies show that people who eat whole carbs, including beans, vegetables, grains, fruit, nuts, and dairy, weigh less, have less abdominal fat, and are generally healthier than those who eat only refined carbs.

But beans beat out other carbs when it comes to weight loss: Legumes, on average, are lower on the glycemic index—a measure of how carbohydrates affect our blood sugar and, consequently, insulin levels—than other foods, including vegetables! How could beans have less of an effect on blood sugar than veggies or oatmeal? Beans contain more fiber, slowing down sugar digestion and its deleterious impact on insulin. What's more, when beans are cooked with a healthy fat like olive oil—hello, Greek diet!—the effect is even more pronounced, with the fat helping to slow down sugar absorption even more.

Here's a look at where beans fall on the glycemic index (GI) compared to other foods. The scale, which measures how foods containing carbohydrates affect blood sugar and insulin, ranges from 0 to over 100, with 0 having no affect and 100 representing pure glucose, a simple sugar. Foods considered low on the GI are those under 55.

White beans = 13
Soybeans = 16
Black beans = 20
Kidney beans = 28
Kale = 32
Broccoli = 32
Skim milk = 32
Apple = 38
Grapes = 46
Mac 'n' cheese = 64
White rice = 69
Whole wheat bread = 71
French fries = 72

GETTING OUT THE GAS

Don't let beans' bad rep for causing flatulence prevent you from losing weight by not loading your plate with this healthy complex carb. Beans cause gas because they contain several types of sugars our bodies can't digest. This isn't a bad thing—these sugars are fermented in the intestine, and the process helps to balance our internal pH. But the offshoot, literally, is gas. You can counter this easily with a few quick tips:

• Gradually increase bean consumption over several weeks.
• Start with canned beans, which contain less indigestible sugars (but wash and drain first to lower sodium content).
• When using dried beans, discard the soaking water and cook the beans in fresh water.
• Drink water to aid digestion and help beans' fiber do its fat-fighting job!

PILLAR FIVE
Seafood (Sensual)

I TRAVELED TO THE SEASIDE CITY OF THESSALONIKI for the first time at the age of eighteen. This is the second biggest metropolis in Greece after Athens, with nearly one million residents today. In Thessaloniki, I went with my friends and family to a small neighborhood called Kalamaria, a scenic place on the coast full of tavernas, many of them famous for their seafood dishes. Until that point in my life, I had never had shellfish. We ordered whatever the server recommended, the freshest seafood they had. They brought out something called *mydopilafo*, a Greek dish full of fresh mussels and rice pilaf, almost like paella. I could smell the aroma before the server even placed the bowl on the table—it was intoxicating, briny yet comforting, almost like the ocean. I was so excited to try something new that I started eating right away, devouring every delicious morsel. The taste of the mydopilafo filled my senses with a salty freshness and the flavor of the mussels. It remains one of the best seafood dishes I've ever tasted.

Today, I make my own version of mydopilafo called *mydia me krokos*. It's based on the dish I had more than thirty-five years ago at that Thessaloniki taverna, but I add Greek saffron. My patrons love this dish, even those who don't like mussels. (To see my recipe for steamed mussels, turn to page 230.)

GROWING UP WITH SEAFOOD

When I was growing up, my family didn't eat a large variety of fresh fish because we weren't close to the ocean—and we didn't have a car. But we did eat salted cod (*vakalao*), smelt (*atherina*), and trout (*pestrofa*). We always had salted cod in our house because it was easy to preserve—we kept it in a box full of salt in the attic, my mother always adding more salt to keep it as fresh as possible. Before we ate it, we would submerge it in water for several hours to flush out the salt, and then cook it with olive oil in a pan or bake it wrapped in a thin phyllo dough crust. This kind of cod pie was delicious and much healthier than how most people eat cod today, breaded and/or deep-fried in unhealthy fats.

My village wasn't near the ocean, but we did have plenty of fish from nearby rivers and lakes. Lake Trichonida is a large lake, almost like the sea, where we would get our smelt. We would cook this fish simply, either roasting it over an open fire or flash-frying it in olive oil, serving either preparation with lots of lemon. In August, during the harvest festival, vendors would skewer pieces of fresh smelt on oregano stems and grill them, the scent traveling all over the village. People would line up to get them. As a young girl, I snuck to the front of the line because I wanted to see how they made them so tasty, and was amazed at the simple and healthy preparation, so different from the fried dough or hot dogs sold at most American fairs and festivals.

Near my village was also the Evinos River, where my father and grandfather would take me swimming while they fished for trout. My father would smoke the trout he caught by building a fire and using a big pot called a *kapnistirio,* which looked like a wok with a rack inside for smoking food. Under the rack, my father placed pieces of wood and then drizzled wine and added herbs like rosemary, pine, and oregano to flavor the wood, which, in turn, infused the smoke. On top of the rack went the fish. My father would smoke it until he could lift up the back of the fish easily with the tip of his knife—that meant it was ready to eat. Today, I still use this trick, but it only works on fish with bones. If the back of the fish lifts up easily with the tip of the knife, it's ready to be served.

SEAFOOD IN ANCIENT GREECE

Look at a map of Greece, and you'll see why seafood was the primary (and sometimes only) animal meat consumed by Greeks for thousands of years. My country has the longest coastline in the Mediterranean, and the eleventh longest coastline in the world, with more than 1,400 islands spread out in the sea. Seafood was easy to catch and common fare in the ancient years, especially for those right on the coast. Most of the fish brought inland was salted (for preservation), but some was transported fresh. The ancient Greeks enjoyed a wide variety of seafood that they caught fresh from the ocean, including sardines, anchovies, red mullet, ray, parrotfish, sturgeon, carp, catfish, yellowfin and bluefin tuna, squid, octopus, eel, sea urchin, and all sorts of shellfish. They would grill or roast seafood over an open fire, often wrapping it first in fig or grapevine leaves, or salt-cure it so they could eat it for days. These methods of preparation made seafood flavorful and healthy, a simple, rich source of protein. And no feast in ancient years was complete without at least one seafood dish.

SEAFOOD FOR WEIGHT LOSS

I eat fish at least three times a week now, something I make sure to do after my experience eating as a Westerner. When I was a jet-setting lobbyist, I stopped eating fish regularly and started consuming a lot of red meat. At first I thought I was just substituting one protein for another, and the red meat would still give me the energy and nutrition I needed. As it turned out, though, all red meat did was make me fat and dull—I gained weight and my hair and skin lost their luster. What I eventually realized is the nutrients in fish, especially omega-3 fats, went far beyond feeding me—they kept me slim and beautiful!

When you have fresh seafood, you need to do very little to make a healthy, nutritious meal. Most seafood you order at fine restaurants is served with just herbs, lemon, and a little fat (olive oil being much healthier than butter). Whenever I go out to new restaurants, I like to order different fish dishes—this way I know I'm getting something healthy and delicious, since most chefs don't need to do much to make fresh seafood taste flavorful and wonderful.

At my restaurants, every fish dish we serve is simple, fresh, and healthy. One of our most popular choices is octopus, even though this is not a popular seafood choice for most Americans. But we've turned many non–octopus eaters into fans of the mollusk. We braise the octopus for a long time until it's tender, and then lightly grill it, serving it with red wine–macerated onions and a touch of *ladolemono*, or lemon–olive oil sauce. (For the recipe, see page 236.) It's so low in calories, yet meaty and delicious, and rich in protein and healthy fat, without heavy animal fat or the chemicals livestock are given today.

SERVING SEAFOOD

Greece is known for its seafood, and as a Greek chef, I've also become known for my seafood dishes. I take great pride in serving only the freshest, most delicious seafood, which is delivered every morning to our kitchens. We inspect every delivery, too, making sure it's straight from the ocean, using all the tips and tricks I learned as a child and over the years as a chef to ensure I have the freshest seafood. And when you have fresh fish, you don't need to do much to make a seafood dish sing. Simple techniques like grilling and pan-searing are best, and you must use delicate sauces to bring out the flavor of the fish rather than hide it. For our seafood recipes, turn to pages 229 to 245.

HOW TO BUY FRESH FISH

FRESH FISH (fillets or whole)

- **Flesh:** The flesh should be firm and resilient. If you press on it, it should bounce back, not leave a mark—if it does, then find another fish.
- **Odor:** This is the big one. Fish shouldn't smell like fish, it should smell briny and like the ocean. If it has a fishy smell, it's a sure sign it's not fresh.
- **Skin:** The skin on the fish should be shiny and metallic looking, not gray, weathered, or dull.
- **Liquid:** If you see liquid near your fish, it should be clear, not milky. If it's milky, your fish is starting to rot.
- **Scales:** If your fish includes scales, make sure they're not flaking off. That means your fish is no longer fresh.

SHELLFISH

- **Lobsters and crabs:** First, make sure they're alive. Then, they must have all their limbs. Finally, the best lobsters and crabs are full of spirit.
- **Mussels, clams, and oysters:** These should also be sold alive. To make sure of this, tap them on their shell—if they close more tightly, they're alive! If they don't or the shell is cracked, choose another batch. After you cook them, throw out any that don't open up during your preparation.
- **Shrimp, squid, and octopus:** It is hard to come by fresh shrimp, squid, and octopus unless you live near the coast. It's better to buy these three frozen, as they keep much better this way.
- **Scallops:** Choose sea and bay scallops that have been dry-packed, not waterlogged or kept in brine, which makes them flavorless and mushy.

PILLAR FIVE
Seafood (Science)

THE BIGGEST COMMON DENOMINATOR of the Mediterranean diet after olive oil is food that actually came out of the Mediterranean Sea—the distinguishing characteristic, after all, of people living along that celestial-blue body of water. Seafood is what made the Mediterranean diet "Mediterranean," so to say, and fish and shellfish more than any other animal meat were the prized game of the ancient Greeks.

As it turns out, the Greeks were on to a good thing: Without a doubt, seafood is the healthiest animal protein you can eat. Not only does eating more fish and shellfish help improve the health of your heart, brain, skin, eyes, and muscles, along with boosting your memory, focus, and longevity, but eating seafood provides the essential fats our bodies *need* to burn fat and lose weight. Without fish, even the best weight-loss efforts will stall. Here's why:

1. SEAFOOD IS THE SINGLE BEST SOURCE OF ESSENTIAL OMEGA-3 FATTY ACIDS YOUR BODY NEEDS TO FIGHT FAT.

Chew on this startling statistic: Ninety-nine percent of Americans don't get enough omega-3 fatty acids. And that's a huge problem, literally, because our dietary lack of this healthy fat is helping make us huge across the country. Omega-3 fatty acids are essential to every single bodily function, including metabolism, hormone regulation, gene regulation, blood-sugar sensitivity, and every other factor that affects our bodies' ability to burn fat. For this reason, studies show that lower levels of omega-3 fatty acids are strongly associated with higher rates of obesity. In fact, a recent study from Iceland found that those who ate cod five times a week lost 4 more pounds on average after 2 months' time than those who consumed a diet with the same number of calories but without any fish!

There are three different types of omega-3 fatty acids: EPA, DHA, and ALA. EPA and DHA are found primarily in seafood like salmon, halibut, tuna, and other foods essential to the Greek diet; ALA is found primarily in plants, like chia, hemp, and flax seeds, nuts, soybeans, and some green leafy vegetables.

Most health benefits associated with omega-3 fatty acids, whether we're talking about improving heart health, revving metabolism, or boosting the body's ability to burn adipose tissue, are associated with EPA and DHA, not ALA. What's more, numerous studies suggest that EPA/DHA supplements, otherwise known as fish oil, and foods fortified with omega-3 fatty acids like eggs and juice, do not activate the same responses in our bodies to the same degree that eating fish does.

So what are the miraculous benefits of EPA and DHA for weight loss? If you eat fish and shellfish at least two times a week, you will reap the following fat-burning benefits:

- Increase your metabolism by as much as 400 calories a day, according to one study from the University of Western Ontario
- Prevent your fat cells from expanding in size, especially around your abdominal area
- Enhance enzymes in your body that help break down stored fat
- Regulate your body's hunger hormone, leptin, which represses cravings and the incidence of binge eating
- Regulate insulin, one of your body's fat-storing hormones
- Boost production of your body's blood sugar–regulating hormone, andiponectin
- Activate gene activity that improves metabolism speed and efficacy
- Reduce gene activity that stimulates the production of new fat cells
- Reduce gene activity that turns baby fat cells into mature fat cells
- Lower your body's levels of chronic inflammation, which is linked to weight gain

Fatty fish like salmon and mackerel have more omega-3s than leaner fish such as tuna. But all types of seafood contains more EPA/DHA omega-3s than any other food, per the following chart:

FOODS HIGHEST IN EPA/DHA OMEGA-3S* (IN MILLIGRAMS)

Atlantic salmon (wild)	1,564
Pink salmon (wild)	1,094
Sockeye salmon (wild)	1,046
Mackerel (canned)	1,046
Rainbow trout	981
Sardines	835
Albacore tuna	733
Sea bass	648
Halibut	395
Oysters	374
Scallops	310
Shrimp	267
Clams	241
Yellowfin tuna	237
Light chunk tuna	230
Fortified egg (1)	150
Cod	134
Mahi-mahi	118
Tilapia	115
Fortified milk (1 cup)	32
Fortified yogurt (4 oz.)	32
Fortified margarine (2 T.)	32

* All amounts based on 3 ounces cooked unless otherwise specified. Data compiled from Colorado State University.

THE WEIGHT-LOSS RATIO: MORE OMEGA-3S, LESS OMEGA-6S

Omega-6s are another essential fatty acid our bodies need to function optimally. But in sharp contrast to omega-3 levels, nearly no one in the West is deficient in omega-6s. Quite the opposite, almost all of us eat way too much omega-6 fat compared to omega-3 fat, causing an imbalance in the body that creates inflammation and leads to weight gain. This is because omega-6s are found in nearly every food common to the Standard American Diet or modern Western way of eating: refined vegetable oils like soy and sunflower, meat, and processed foods like cookies, crackers, and fast food. Studies show consuming omega-6 fatty acids in the quantities most Americans and Europeans do without a commensurate amount of omega-3s has helped fuel the Western world's obesity epidemic. The only way to right the balance is to reduce your intake of omega-6s by limiting consumption of refined cooking oils (another reason to reach for olive oil!) and processed foods and increasing your intake of omega-3s by eating more fish.

2. SEAFOOD IS LOWER IN CALORIES, SATURATED FAT, AND CHOLESTEROL THAN OTHER ANIMAL PROTEIN.

Ounce for ounce, seafood is generally lower in calories than red meat and chicken. Lean selections like cod, flounder, sole, and shellfish contain approximately 100 calories for a 3-ounce cooked serving—70 calories less than chicken breast and 20 calories less than skinless chicken breast. American fast-food restaurants like to bread and fry low-fat fish, as they do with chicken, but Greek chefs and gourmands alike know lean seafood (and poultry) is a delicacy that tastes best when grilled, baked, broiled, or stir-fried with the right spices, herbs, and healthy oils.

Fattier fish like salmon has more calories—150 per 3-ounce cooked serving—but they also have more fat-fighting omega-3s and, on average, slightly more protein. What's more, you're still racking up significant calorie savings by eating fattier fish instead of red meat or pork, to the tune of nearly 100 calories when you compare a salmon fillet to a beef burger you might get at a restaurant. Finally, fattier fish are often the lowest-calorie entrées to choose from when eating out since they're rarely served with anything but a little olive oil or butter—not the rich sauces and gravies usually served with red meat, pork, and even poultry.

It's important to remember that losing weight isn't just about calories. Our bodies need fat to burn fat, and a low-fat diet is *not* an effective (or satisfying!) way to lose weight. But not all fat is created equal, as discussed in Pillar One: Olive Oil. Saturated fat, found in animal meat and products like butter and cream, along with processed snacks like potato chips, won't help you burn fat—eating too much will help you gain weight instead. Interesting new research from American University's Center for Behavioral Neuroscience found that consuming a diet high in saturated fat stimulates changes in the brain that fuel overconsumption of the same types of food. Another 8-year study of more than 41,000 women found that a diet high in monounsaturated fat (found in olive oil) and polyunsaturated fat (found in seafood) did not cause weight gain, while a diet rich in saturated fat from animal meats and processed foods caused significant weight gain.

Another benefit to seafood is that it's lower in heart-clogging cholesterol than red meat and skin-on chicken. While this won't help you directly lose weight, eating less LDL ("bad") cholesterol by substituting seafood for red meat and fattier poultry when possible can help reduce your risk for heart disease, stroke, metabolic syndrome, and other cardiovascular illness. (Note that shrimp and squid are higher in cholesterol than other seafood—if you have high cholesterol, consider other options with less cholesterol from the following chart.)

HOW SEAFOOD STACKS UP TO ANIMAL MEAT

Food (3 oz. serving)	Calories	Total Fat (G)	Sat. Fat (G)	Cholesterol (MG)	Protein (G)
Oysters	50	1	0	20	4
Shrimp	85	1	0	165	18
Cod	90	1	0	50	19
Flounder	100	1.5	0	60	21
Filet of sole	100	1.5	0	60	20
Halibut	120	2	0	35	23
Chicken breast, skinless	120	1.5	0	70	24
Salmon	150	7	1.5	55	23
Chicken breast, skin on	170	7	2	70	21
Beef sirloin steak	170	6	2	75	25
Beef tenderloin	180	9	3	70	26
Lamb chop	180	3	3	80	24
Pork loin	190	8	3	25	25
Ground beef, 90% lean	190	10	4	70	22
Ground beef, 80% lean (average)	230	15	6	80	22

FIGHT BAD HEALTH WITH GOOD SEAFOOD

A slimmer, trimmer you isn't the only reason to up your intake of seafood and the marine-based omega-3 fatty acids that come along with it. Studies show that eating the EPA and DHA fats found in fish can reduce your risk of almost every major health condition, from heart disease, diabetes, and certain cancers to asthma, arthritis, depression, ADHD, Alzheimer's, inflammatory bowel disease, osteoporosis, even dermatitis and premature aging.

Studies show that eating just 1 or 2 servings of fish per week can reduce your risk of dying from heart disease by an incredible 36 percent. Meanwhile, large-scale research from China of 900,000 women found that those who ate the most omega-3 fats from fish were 14 percent less likely to develop breast cancer. Countless other studies show similar effects from omega-3s on a host of other diseases and health conditions—far too many to list here—simply by eating more fish.

Finally, fish won't just make you healthier and thinner, it can also make you look younger. Because omega-3s help reduce free radicals that can wreak havoc on skin, increasing your consumption also slows the physical signs of aging, like wrinkles and loose skin, while easing symptoms of rosacea, psoriasis, and other skin conditions.

THE TRUTH ABOUT TOXINS IN SEAFOOD

It's an unfortunate circumstance that would appall the seafaring and sea-loving ancient Greeks: Today's oceans are polluted with a number of toxins, including mercury and PCBs. Those toxins are now found in fish, even those that are caught in the wild. But the benefits of eating seafood far outweigh the risks, especially if you choose smart seafood. Most of us know that wild-caught salmon is significantly lower in PCBs than farmed salmon. But some farmed varieties, like trout and bass, are fine to eat. In general, small fish like anchovies and sardines contain fewer toxins (and more omega-3s) than large fish like tuna and sea bass. Tuna can be high in mercury, but canned chunk light tuna is lower in the heavy metal than canned albacore tuna. Choose domestically raised tilapia over that imported from Asia. The only seafood you should avoid eating due to toxin content are mackerel, swordfish, tilefish, marlin, orange roughy, and bigeye and ahi tuna. For more information or to download a free app or pocket guide on safe seafood choices, visit the Monterey Bay Aquarium's Seafood Watch Program at www.montereybayaquarium .org/cr/seafoodwatch.aspx.

Whole Grains (Sensual)

ALL OF MY LIFE, I never feared bread. The Atkins diet always seemed like such a ridiculous concept to me—to eliminate a basic food group from your diet and one of the three greats in the Mediterranean triad (olive oil, wheat, and wine). For Greeks, bread is an essential part of how we eat.

I'll admit, I did try a low-carb diet once. I lasted four days. It started out the way any diet starts out—full of hope and promise. Quickly though, I noticed my resolve wavering. At first, I thought it was just my mind craving my favorite foods because I had been conditioned all my life to enjoy bread, pasta, and grains. But by the second day, I felt my body itching for things, not because I wanted these foods, but because I *needed* them. Still, I tried to stick with the diet, filling myself with red meat, processed protein bars, and salads. My mood worsened and I began getting terrible headaches, yet I continued to tell myself my body would get used to this new way of eating.

On day three, I had a business meeting and almost ruined a major deal because I appeared dull and miserable—for me, this was the beginning of the end. That night, I decided to weigh myself. I couldn't believe the scale—I had gained a pound! My body was rebelling against this way of eating as much as my mind was. I thought, "Why would anyone put himself or herself through this voluntarily?" I would have stopped the diet that night, but I had already given away all the bread and pasta in my house. The next morning, though, I went to the market, bought myself some whole-grain pita bread, and savored the carbs. I knew in that moment, as a wave of calm came over me, that the ancient Greeks had it right—bread and grains were essential, a necessary part of any diet. To remove these food groups completely made no sense, regardless of how strong anyone's desire was to be thin.

WHOLE GRAINS IN ANCIENT GREECE

The ancient Greeks consumed so much olive oil, wine, and wheat that these three foods are commonly referred to as the Mediterranean triad. But the type of wheat the Greeks ate wasn't like what most Westerners consume today in processed and packaged breads, rolls, crackers, and cereals. In ancient times, the only grains that existed were whole grains, primarily whole wheat and whole barley. The Greeks made gruel from whole wheat and also ground the crop for flour. With barley, they cooked it like we do with rice and other whole grains, and roasted it before grinding it into flour.

Both these flours were used to make bread, the primary food of ancient Greece. The Greeks served bread dipped in olive oil or wine with meals and also used it as a utensil to scoop up whatever food was served with it. The foods that accompanied bread were referred to as *opson*, or relish.

Another way grains were consumed in the ancient times was in the form of something called *kykeon*, similar to a modern-day smoothie. This was made by combining barley gruel and water with different herbs and sometimes cheese, honey, and wine, as well.

GROWING UP WITH WHOLE GRAINS

My favorite mornings growing up were when my whole family was together. On those special days, my father would make us kykeon, just like the ancient Greeks drank. He liked to make it with mint, thyme, and a little bit of honey, and at the last moment before he gave it to us, he'd mix in some of my mother's yogurt. We drank this before school, and it made me feel strong and satisfied all day. I liked it not only for the taste, but because it made me feel connected to my heritage, like an ancient goddess!

Whole grains usually brought the whole family together. We grew wheat, corn, barley, and many other grains on my farm. My brother and I would take our family's donkey, Mendis, and bring the grains from our house to the *mylos,* the village mill. This was something I loved to do because there was this earthy aroma that reminded me of my grandmother, and I got to be a part of the culinary process from start to finish.

When we returned from the mill with the freshly ground grains, my grandmother and Aunt

Maria would get to work right away, making dough for bread and pasta. They baked bread in an oven we kept outside, and its intoxicating scent traveled all over our house and across our farm. They also made lots of different types of homemade pasta, some of which would be dried and saved to eat over the year.

We ate pasta about three times a week, often for Sunday dinner. My favorite dish was orzo pasta, or *kritharaki,* with vegetables and chicken, although about once a month we had it with lamb. The Monday after this meal was my best day of the week, because I felt very strong, healthy, and balanced.

WHOLE GRAINS TODAY

Growing up, there was no such thing as refined flours or grains—we only had what Americans now call whole grains. After trying a low-carb diet only to gain weight, I decided to start paying attention to the quality of the carbs I was eating, returning to the whole-grain breads and pastas of my childhood. I noticed a difference right away. I didn't feel sluggish, tired, or bloated, but clean, thin, and full of energy. I began to wonder why people were eating refined grains in the first place. Why would you choose to eat something that wasn't good for you *and* made you gain weight? I also realized why many dieters would attempt to stop eating carbs—of course, they thought carb-rich grains were making them fat because all they knew and were consuming were fattening refined grains!

When you discover whole grains, a whole new world opens up. When I came to New York, I discovered a different and exciting world of grains. At first, I admit, the idea of eating something like quinoa, which is not a Greek food at all, went against my "grain," but then I thought about it. One of the biggest underlying tenets of Greek cuisine is to use whatever is sustainable and available—and quinoa fits that description. The healthy whole grain also is high in fiber, high in protein, and gluten-free, so it's filling and versatile no matter what diet you follow. And while these are great qualities, what really sold me on it was the texture. Slightly chewy, but still flavorful and soft, all at the same time—a chef's dream!

I use many different grains like quinoa, farro, barley, and rice, serving them as main and side dishes, both cold and hot. I like to think of them all as blank canvases on which to express my culinary creativity. For example, I use farro to make a risotto-style dish with wild mushrooms, onions, vegetables, herbs, and vegetable stock. But I also like to toast farro in the oven and use it as a garnish for seafood and salads to add texture.

To me, there is nothing better than homemade whole-grain pasta. I serve it at my restaurant, made with whole-grain farro and wheat. It has become so popular, in fact, that I recently started selling my pasta under the brand name Loi, which is now distributed in supermarkets nationwide.

Whole Grains (Science)

BREAD, PASTA, GRAINS, and any food made with flour: All have been falsely maligned for causing weight gain. But the truth is, our bodies need bread and other healthy whole grains to lose weight, just like we need healthy fat to burn fat. Try to drop pounds without eating the right grains and not only will you make yourself miserable and irritable, you can also sabotage your metabolism and hormone function to the point of no return, causing your weight-loss efforts to stall and even triggering weight gain.

The ancient Greek diet was heavy on carbs, including whole-grain bread, but the ancient Greeks themselves boasted a leaner shape than today's bread-eating Americans. Why? The grains and bread the ancient Greeks consumed were remarkably different from what's sold on store shelves and offered in restaurants today. Just like not all fats are created equal when it comes to weight loss, not all grains and flours will help you drop pounds. Quite the opposite. Choose the wrong type—refined flours, processed grains, or products made with them (the majority of what's available on supermarket shelves)—and you will gain weight. Here is what you need to know about eating the right type of grains to get thin:

1. YOUR BODY NEEDS THE COMPLEX CARBS IN WHOLE GRAINS TO LOSE WEIGHT AND FUNCTION PROPERLY.

Forget everything you've heard about low-carb diets. Simply put, cutting carbs from your diet is not an effective, sustainable, or healthy way to lose weight. The truth is, our bodies need carbs from bread, pasta, and grains to fuel our hearts, brains, and muscles, as well as the immune system and every other major body function. Complex carbs are our main energy source, and every major world health institution, including the Institute of Medicine, recommends getting anywhere from 45 percent to 65 percent of your daily calories from complex carbs—even if you're trying to lose weight! Yes, you can get complex carbs from vegetables and fruit, too, but grains are the best source, and without consuming foods like orzo, quinoa, bread, and oatmeal, it's almost impossible to get enough complex carbs to keep all your body's systems—including your metabolism—running at optimal levels.

For this reason, nearly every major study shows that people who eat more healthy complex carbs like whole-grain bread, pasta, and cereal lose more weight than people who don't. One of the most significant research efforts to demonstrate this was a Canadian study of more than 4,500 people that found that those who ate the most carbs were significantly thinner than those who ate the fewest. In fact, researchers concluded that people looking to stay slim should get up to a whopping 64 percent of their daily calorie intake from carbs like whole-grain bread and pasta.

2. THE MORE WHOLE GRAINS AND THE FEWER REFINED GRAINS YOU CONSUME, THE MORE WEIGHT YOU'LL LOSE.

A loaf of bread on the supermarket shelf can help you lose weight—or possibly cause you to pack on extra pounds. Yep, that's how big of a difference there is between food made with whole grains and food made with refined grains.

What are refined grains? And what's so bad about them, anyway? All grains—common grains like wheat, corn, oats, rye, and rice, and less common grains such as spelt, amaranth, farro, and quinoa—start out as whole kernels made up of three layers: an outer bran, an inner germ, and an inner filler, the endosperm. When food manufacturers refine a grain to turn it into a product like bread, rolls, pasta, or cereal, they strip the bran and germ out of the grain's kernel, leaving only the filler, the endosperm. This process removes most of the grain's fiber, along with important B vitamins, iron, and other micronutrients that help increase satiety, aid metabolism, and slow digestion. Without fiber and micronutrients, refined grains are, essentially, empty calories, nutrient-devoid food. Compounding that fact, many store-bought breads, crackers, pastas, cereals, and other refined grain products include added sugars, unhealthy fats, preservatives, bleach oxidizers, and other toxins that can interfere with your body's metabolism, hormones, and overall well-being.

Whole grains, and the foods made from them, are never refined, so they include all three parts of the kernel—bran, germ, and endosperm—along with all the naturally occurring nutrients that come with them. Whole grains can be cracked, crushed, rolled, or cooked, but these processes don't strip the kernel of its fiber or micronutrients. Since whole grains are plants, too, they act similarly to vegetables, fruits, beans, and nuts in your body, working overtime by delivering fiber, protein, water, vitamins, minerals, antioxidants, and other micronutrients to fill you up while keeping your metabolism running at full speed.

Research shows eating whole grains can help decrease the risk of heart disease, diabetes, cancer, and other chronic illness. Similarly, countless studies show people who consume more whole grains weigh less and have a healthier body mass index (BMI) than those who don't. Research also shows people who eat several servings of whole grains daily while limiting their intake of refined grains have less belly fat.

ALL THESE ARE UNREFINED GRAIN PRODUCTS:
- Amaranth
- Barley
- Buckwheat
- **Corn,** including whole cornmeal and popcorn
- Millet
- **Oats,** including quick-cooking and rolled oats
- **Quinoa,** including white, red, and black
- **Rice,** including brown rice and colored rice
- Rye
- **Sorghum** (also called milo)
- Teff
- Triticale
- **Whole wheat,** including spelt, emmer, farro, einkorn, Kamut, durum, bulgur, cracked wheat, and wheatberries
- Wild rice

UNREFINED GRAIN PRODUCTS:
- White flour
- All-purpose flour
- Whole wheat flour
- Sourdough
- Stone-ground wheat

- Enriched wheat flour
- White rice
- White pasta
- Matzo
- Oat and wheat bran
- Degerminated cornmeal
- Wheat germ
- Corn flakes

HOW TO SPOT A WHOLE GRAIN—AND AVOID REFINED IMPOSTERS

Most packaged foods and snacks contain a refined grain or flour. But it's easy to be fooled by healthy sounding labels like "multigrain," "stone-ground," "100 percent wheat," or "organic"—*none* of which indicates the food you're buying, whether it's bread, crackers, pasta, or cereal, is made from whole grains. The only way to be sure you're getting whole grains is to check the ingredients label. The grain, whether wheat, corn, oats, or another type, must include the word "whole" to be, in fact, a whole grain—for example, "whole oats," "whole corn," "whole wheat," or "stoneground whole wheat." Exceptions to this rule are brown rice, wheatberries, and oats (including quick-cooking and old-fashioned rolled oats). You can also look for products that feature the 100% Whole Grain Stamp, given only to products that feature whole grains.

3. PLEASURE FACTOR ALERT: EATING WHOLE-GRAIN CARBS MAKES US HAPPY, AND HAPPY MAKES US THIN.

There's actually a scientific reason why bread and pasta are called "comfort foods:" Our bodies and brains need these starchy complex carbs for happy and healthy mood levels. If you've ever tried cutting bread, pasta, cereal, and other grains from your diet, you know what we're talking about: the feelings of irritation, lethargy, and even depression that come from depriving your body of the lasting energy it needs. And the effect isn't due to the fact that you're upset that you can't have a slice of warm bread or a bowl of macaroni and cheese: Complex carbs like those in grains, bread, and pasta are necessary for our brains to produce the body's primary mood-boosting hormone, serotonin. Without the carbs from these foods, our hormone levels plunge dangerously low, sending us into a funk that makes it nearly impossible to exercise or retain any healthy eating or lifestyle plan. This is a big reason researchers have found for people giving up on low-carb diets before they can see results: They simply don't have enough serotonin to feel like doing anything worthwhile, including eating or acting healthfully. What's more, studies show people often *gain* weight after following a low-carb diet. One reason for this is that you begin to crave high-sugar foods like cookies, cakes, and packaged breads in the hope that their refined carbs can turn around your plummeting outlook on life. But quite the opposite, refined carbs don't have the same effect on mood as healthy whole grains do. Instead, they spike our bodies' blood-sugar levels so much, the resulting insulin surge makes our energy and mood levels plunge, causing weight gain.

THE SECRET TO WEIGHT LOSS WITH WHOLE GRAINS: OLIVE OIL

The ancient Greeks unknowingly adhered to an effective slimming habit by pairing fresh bread with olive oil before most meals. The combination of this healthy antioxidant-rich fat with high-fiber whole grains has been shown to significantly increase satiety, slowing the movement of food through the body while making it less likely we'll overeat at lunch or dinner—or during the dangerous after-dinner hours. Even Dr. Oz recommends eating whole-grain bread with olive oil before meals, saying the combination is one of the best ways to reduce the amount of food we eat during and after meals.

Wine (Sensual)

WINE IS AN OBJECT near to my heart—and good for it! I believe strongly in its magical powers, not just for my health, but also for its ability to bring people together, to transform ingredients, and to enhance life. Greece has an incredible wine culture, and when I opened my restaurant, I wanted to bring to New York City not only the food of my people, but our wine, as well. But getting Americans to accept Greek wine was a bit of a hurdle, with many customers arguing the Italians and the French have a better selection. This surprised me. Did these wine enthusiasts not know the Greeks helped to invent the wine trade? And how can you eat the food of a nation and not pair it with the wine of that country? Wine is integral to what we call the Mediterranean triad: wine, wheat, and olive oil, the three most important ingredients in our cuisine. I decided that educating my customers was something I simply had to do.

WINE CULTURE IN ANCIENT GREECE

The ancient Greeks believed wine was a gift from the gods, so important to human life and health that one of the twelve Olympic gods was named after the drink—Dionysus, the god of wine, wine-making, and the grape harvest. There were festivals held in his honor, celebrating all that he represented, as well as the importance of wine as a trade commodity.

The ancients drank up to two glasses of red wine a day, but they consumed wine differently than we do today. The style of wine in ancient times was most commonly sweet and aromatic, flavored with herbs and flowers, though there were drier wines as well. Wine was almost always diluted with water, which was a mark of civilized behavior—most ancients believed only barbarians drank *akratos* (unmixed wine).

Wine was also used as a panacea, functioning as an antiseptic, a cure for fevers, an analgesic, a diuretic, a tonic, and as a digestive aid. And while the ancient Greeks revered wine and drank it daily, they also understood the downsides to excessive wine consumption, alluding in ancient literature to hangovers or even death.

The One Thing the Greeks Got Wrong

No society is 100 percent perfect, and one thing the Greeks got wrong is that they did not approve of women consuming wine for anything other than therapeutic or medicinal purposes. The ancients believed wine made women fertile to a point, but also had the ability to induce abortions. But on this particular subject, I disagree with the opinion of my ancestors. Wine (in moderation) is excellent for women!

WINE IN MY YOUTH

Believe it or not, wine was part of my life from a very young age. We made our own wine at home from our family's vineyard, where we grew black and white grapes. I loved to wander into the vineyard and pick grapes, often sucking the insides right out of the skin. During the harvest, our donkey, Mendis (he, too, was my friend), would carry large bundles of grapes home on his back. Winemaking was a joyous affair in our village, and everyone helped. The strongest men in our village would come to our house and help us pour the bundles of grapes into a large wooden wine vat the size of three men—every house had its own wine vat to crush grapes. I would climb into the vat on the ladder with my friends and siblings, and we would all stomp on the grapes. This was one of our favorite forms of exercise, jumping up and down on the sweet grapes, and I remember feeling drunk with joy just from their scent. I loved the stains the grapes would leave on our feet, a reddish-purple badge of honor I wore with pride. I tried to make the stains last as long as it took for the wine to ferment, or about one month.

My grandmother always said wine was full of antioxidants, and good for all kinds of ailments, including indigestion and poor circulation. My grandfather gave us bread dipped in wine and unfermented grape juice for breakfast before school, a simple meal that gave us strength for the rest of the day. During the colder months, we would toast our bread in the fireplace and then dip it in the wine.

In my house, all the adults had a daily glass of wine—everyone knew it was important for their hearts and health. In the months without an R (May, June, July, and August), my parents would add water to their wine to dilute it, the way the ancients did. They did this because they believed one needed the full warming power of wine without water in the winter months. But during the summer, mixing water with wine prevented the alcohol from sapping their energy.

WINE IN MY LIFE

I didn't begin drinking wine until my twenties, even though in Greece it is normal to drink at a much younger age than in the United States. Moderation has always been preached, and when I was growing up, there weren't any town drunks where we lived.

When I left Greece and began traveling, I was exposed to a world of wine outside Greece. I tasted different grapes and varietals that I'd never had—it was a whole new oenophilic world for me! Though I enjoyed both reds and whites, I felt a kindred spirit with the reds, especially *xinomavro*, a type of Greek grape that reminded me of my childhood wine-stomping adventures. I began to experiment not only with wines, but with the foods that were supposed to pair with them. But as I adopted more Western ways of eating, I also found myself no longer following the ancient wisdom of *metron ariston*, "everything in moderation," when it came to wine.

It was only after my great Greek friend Dr. Nikolaides, who helped me lose forty pounds, reminded me of the importance of olive oil that I remembered wine's place in the Mediterranean triad (wheat, wine, olive oil). As I stopped eating according to the Western style, I also moved back toward the Greek style of drinking, consuming no more than two glasses of wine a day. Quickly, I noticed a positive reaction from my body, a shrinking reaction. Today, I still drink a glass of wine daily. Toward the end of the night, you can usually find me sitting at a table, with a glass of wine, surrounded by friends, and a platter of food to share. You can hear the laughter, smell the food, and feel the sense of community. For me, this is what life is all about.

COOKING WITH WINE

If you've never had Greek wine, you cannot call yourself a true oenophile. There are more than 300 grape varieties indigenous to Greece, and many harken back to ancient times. The climate and soil in Greece produce distinct grapes, and the result is dozens of unique varietals that taste like nothing else in the world.

I don't believe in using low-quality wine for cooking. Although some chefs think you don't need a premium wine to make sauces and dishes, I think the quality of every one of your ingredients affects the quality of your food. I make it a point to cook only with wines I'd be willing to drink, and wine is a common ingredient in many of my dishes, important to braising chicken and other meats and making sauces for everything from vegetables and seafood to pasta and fruit desserts. In fact, I use both red and white to cook many foods I don't grill, including my famous *kokoras krassato*, the Greek version of coq au vin.

_____ TIPS AND TRICKS FOR COOKING WITH WINE_____

- Choose wines made from a blend of grapes when making sauces—avoid those aged in oak.
- Cook sauces with wine slowly over a low heat, just below a simmer.
- Don't throw out the wine left over from cooking! Instead, freeze it in ice trays to use the next time a recipe calls for wine.

PILLAR SEVEN
Wine (Science)

WHY WOULD ANYONE want to give up hot summer nights with a glass of cold, crisp Chardonnay? Or cozy winter afternoons with a smooth, rich Shiraz? On the Greek Diet, you don't have to sacrifice things like wine that we think make life worth living. In fact, we encourage you to drink a glass or two every day. By doing so, not only will you be adopting a truly Mediterranean diet, you'll also improve your overall health and speed your weight-loss efforts.

Undoubtedly, you've already heard about wine's amazing health benefits. The oldest alcoholic beverage in the world, wine has been shown to help lower the risk of heart attack and stroke, increase cognitive function, ward off diabetes, even thwart certain types of cancer. With such powerful effects, why wouldn't the drink also influence our bodies' metabolism and fat-burning capabilities?

Recent research shows moderate wine consumption helps curb cravings, increases metabolism, and prevents long-term weight gain. Simply put, people who enjoy a daily glass or two of wine are significantly thinner—and healthier—than those who abstain. Surprised? Anthropologists and historians aren't. Since humans began drinking wine some 7,000 years ago, cultures that have consumed the fermented grape juice, like the ancient Greeks, have historically had lower rates of obesity and chronic disease than those who have not. As research shows—and the ancient Greeks proved—drinking wine increases our enjoyment of what we eat and stimulates pleasure centers in the brain that make losing weight and keeping it off a more sustainable and pleasant process.

1. WINE HAS SPECIFIC PROPERTIES THAT INCREASE METABOLISM AND HELP YOUR BODY BURN FAT.

If major pharmaceutical manufacturers could figure out a way to turn wine's good properties into a diet drug, they would. That's because an overwhelming amount of research shows resveratrol, the leading healthy antioxidant in wine, has amazing effects on our metabolism and fat cells, not to mention our overall health. A recent study published in the journal *Cell Metabolism* found that resveratrol triggers healthy changes to our energy metabolism that allow us to burn more calories, even at rest! The effect is so pronounced that it increases your caloric burn for a full hour and a half after you finish a glass.

Resveratrol doesn't just work wonders on your metabolism. Scientists have also found that it helps lower levels of blood sugar and insulin, reduces fat storage in our liver, improves cell function, and significantly decreases any overall bodily inflammation. What's more, studies show these benefits work while we sleep, suggesting this fat-burning wine antioxidant bumps up the body's overall efficiency.

But you can't just pop a supplement with resveratrol (yes, they do exist) and expect all the stomach-slimming benefits inherent in a glass of Merlot. A number of studies have concluded that wine stimulates weight loss. For example, an impressive 13-year study of nearly 20,000 women found that those who drank a glass or two of wine a day were 30 percent less likely to be overweight than nondrinkers. While the correlation was also noted for women who drank beer and liquor, the effect was far more pronounced among those who consumed wine, particularly red wine. Furthermore, research has found wine drinkers have narrower waists and less belly fat than liquor drinkers. What's more, a fascinating study published in the *Journal of Biological Chemistry* found that a chemical in wine called piceatannol, which is unrelated to resveratrol, actually blocks the growth of fat cells.

Metron Ariston

We repeat this Greek phrase throughout the book, but when it comes to wine, "everything in moderation" couldn't be more important. We encourage you to enjoy one or two 5-ounce glasses of wine per night—nothing more. Having more can seriously jeopardize your health and weight-loss efforts. What's more, if you have a preexisting health condition or are taking any prescription medications, talk to your doctor before increasing your intake of wine or any alcohol.

---

2. THE ALCOHOL IN WINE IS A POWERFUL ANTIDOTE TO WEIGHT GAIN.

Wine has special and specific properties that help us lose weight. But research also shows that drinking alcohol of any kind, including beer and hard liquor, helps us manage our weight, suggesting that there's something about alcohol itself that acts as a powerful antidote to weight gain. Perhaps one of the most significant studies to point scientists toward this conclusion was a groundbreaking research effort that included more than 19,000 women at the Brigham and Women's Hospital in Boston. Scientists there deduced that women who drank a moderate amount of alcohol every day over the 13 years of the study didn't gain as much weight as those who avoided drinking altogether, or, conversely, those who drank heavily. The weight difference between the groups of women was significant, too, with teetotalers gaining 6 more pounds on average than those who enjoyed one or two drinks per day.

While impressive, the Brigham and Women's study hasn't been the only one to show alcohol prevents weight gain. Another study of 50,000 women over 8 years published in the journal *Obesity Research* also concluded moderate drinkers didn't gain as much weight as those who drank heavily or didn't drink at all.

But why would drinking alcohol prevent weight gain? Wouldn't the extra calories lead to more pounds? The answer is surprising. First, alcohol triggers a thermogenic response in the body, meaning it increases heart rate and, in turn, revs up metabolism. Think about it. Do you ever feel warmer after a cocktail? That's alcohol's thermogenic response at work, boosting your heart rate and metabolism. The effect lasts up to ninety minutes after one drink, allowing any wine you have with dinner to help you actually burn the calories of that meal.

Alcohol's diet-friendly effects go beyond metabolism, too—the drink also affects our outlook on life . . . and food. Research has found that women who drink alcoholic beverages consume less sugar, in part because alcohol lights up the brain's pleasure center. Having a drink at dinner or out with friends provides a sense of contentment that helps fulfill our need for sweets and other high-calorie foods. If a heart-healthy 120-calorie glass of wine satisfies the body's pleasure receptors, it's a smarter choice than an artery-clogging 500-calorie slice of cheesecake.

All this exciting research does come with a few caveats. First, research that shows alcohol can help prevent weight gain is based on moderate drinking only—that means one to two drinks per day. Second, studies suggest, as anecdotal experience can corroborate, that people can make poor food choices when drinking, since alcohol lowers inhibition and self-control. If you tend to do so after a drink or two, curtail the effect by consuming wine only with meals and limiting your intake to just one glass.

3. WINE INCREASES YOUR PLEASURE IN FOOD AND LIFE AS YOU LOSE WEIGHT.

The famous Greek playwright Euripides said, "When there is no wine, there is no love." Thousands of years later, we couldn't agree more. Drinking wine with family, friends, and loved ones is one of life's greatest pleasures, and no diet should force you to forsake sharing that social experience. Weight-loss plans that expect you to go to family dinners, after-work functions, holiday celebrations, and parties without having a glass of wine are setting you up for a miserable time—and, ultimately, failure, because those diets aren't socially sustainable. In comparison, on the Greek Diet, you can enjoy a glass of wine out with friends or family and feel good about yourself, knowing you're helping to meet your weight-loss goals.

A glass of wine with dinner can also make the dinner itself a more satisfying experience. For example, what sounds like a more pleasurable meal: Salmon with greens and water, or salmon with greens and red wine? Studies show when we make the most of our meals, by drinking wine, lighting candles, and sitting down with family or friends, we're more likely to feel full and satisfied—and less likely to eat later—than when we don't take the time to turn our meals into memorable experiences.

Another way wine can speed weight loss is by enhancing the flavor of food. It's no mystery that wine helps bring out individual ingredients in a meal—the reason wine pairing today has turned into a multibillion-dollar industry for restaurants and oenophiles. Better yet, when you use wine to increase your enjoyment of food, it makes meals taste better, leaving you, once again, more satisfied and less likely to overeat or give into cravings.

Lastly, the Greek Diet isn't a temporary weight-loss plan. As research shows, quick-fix diets don't work because they don't teach you to eat right, instead letting you regain any weight you lost the minute you return to normal eating. On the Greek Diet, we teach you to eat a new normal now, with plenty of wine, olive oil, and other pleasurable foods that you could never give up for good, so you can continue to look and feel good for life.

Herbs and Spices (Sensual)

THE CUISINE OF MY PEOPLE relies heavily on herbs and spices—without them, the world would be boring and bland. For me, the fragrance, flavor, and color of herbs and spices make every food taste and look better. Certain herbs, like oregano and mint, speak to my soul with their amazing qualities, medicinal properties, and culinary flexibility. These two herbs remind me of my past—and excite me when I think about how I can use them in the future. But all herbs and spices make me excited because they have the power to make every food they touch healthier, more flavorful, and more filling.

ANCIENT GREECE

In ancient years, only select herbs like mint, rosemary, and thyme were used for food, but spices pervaded many dishes. One of the world's most expensive spices today, saffron, grew natively in ancient Greece and was used in many dishes, along with *mahalebi,* a popular spice with a bark-like flavor. Perhaps the most commonly used spice was anise, which also grew in ancient Greece, and added a deep licorice flavor to cooked and baked foods. Wealthier families bought imported cinnamon, cumin, black pepper, cloves, and other spices, and used them to impress their guests at social functions. And anise, pine, and other herbs were used by ancient Greeks to flavor wine and water.

Herbs and spices were also used extensively for medicinal purposes, so much so that many herbal remedies now make up the basis of many modern pharmaceuticals. Hippocrates, often called the father of modern medicine, prescribed a variety of different herbs to treat many common illnesses, using ginger to treat cold symptoms, rosemary to cure a nasty headache, and garlic to lower high blood pressure.

CULINARY HERBS AND SPICES

When I was growing up, the beautiful aromas from herbs and spices filled my family's house. Fresh herbs like mint, basil, thyme, dill, and rosemary all grew wild on my family's land, and we picked many of them right off the plant to cook and use as medicine. To get oregano, we had to hike up into the mountains, where it grew wild. We would pick it fresh and then dry it under the hot sun to use later in food and as a palliative for all types of ailments. But oregano was the only herb we used dry, because it had a more exciting flavor this way.

My grandmother baked with cinnamon, cardamom, cloves, nutmeg, and allspice, and used cinnamon in many of our savory dishes, as well. Greek saffron, or *krokos,* was a prized possession in our household because it was expensive. Aunt Maria used it sparingly when cooking beans, fish, and many of her other signature dishes, and we always knew it was going to be a fantastic meal when we saw the vibrant red threads soaking in water or milk. My sense of smell played an important role in my early life, and I always knew whether I would like something based on its smell. Anise's sharp licorice scent was one of the only smells and flavors I grew into; I disliked it as a child, but grew to love it as I got older.

My grandmother and Aunt Maria, the two main cooks in our house, taught me the value of restraint in cooking. They told me that you could always add more, but once you add too much, you can't take it back—this lesson was especially true about fundamental seasonings like salt and pepper. They taught me that there are proper times to add different ingredients—certain spices were better added in the beginning or middle of cooking to build layers of flavor, while most fresh herbs should be included at the end, so you don't lose their delicate flavor, bright color, and naturally occurring nutrients.

MY FAMILY'S HERBAL HOMEOPATHY

My grandmother might as well have been a doctor—she had a cure for everything when I was growing up! But she didn't develop these cures on her own; her medicinal knowledge was passed down to her from generations before, all the way back to our ancient ancestors. Whenever something was wrong, she knew exactly what to do, and it always involved an herb or spice. Here are some of her traditional treatments:

- **Upset stomach:** As a child, I was full of energy, but sometimes it was nervous energy and my stomach would get upset. When this happened, my grandmother gave me a tea made from fresh mint or chamomile that calmed my stomach down immediately.
- **Eye infection:** For eye infections, my grandmother soaked cotton balls in chamomile tea and made us rest with them on our eyelids. The next morning, we were good as new! Many people still do this today, preferring this method to prescription ointments.
- **Insect bites:** We would prevent mosquito bites with basil plants. My grandmother put them all over our house, inside and out, to repel the bugs.
- **Headaches:** My grandmother also prescribed fresh basil (in tea or food) to cure headaches.
- **Concentration:** In ancient times, they used to make a crown out of rosemary sprigs to help calm headaches and clear the mind, especially when studying. My grandmother taught me this, and I always did it while preparing for exams.
- **Sinus problems:** Oregano was my grandmother's go-to for everything—to make things taste better, smell beautiful, and, if we ever had problems with our sinuses (aside from the time I ruined the cucumbers), we would make a tea out of it and drink it.

HERBS AND SPICES FOR WEIGHT LOSS

One of the reasons I gained so much weight as a businesswoman in my thirties was because I was eating so much Americanized fast food, much of which was bland and boring. There was very little flavor in the food, other than salt, fat, and sugar, and I found myself overeating to try to feel satisfied with the taste. Where were the pungent seasonings that gave foods such wonderful spiciness and flavor? When I returned to eating a traditional Greek diet and started making my own food, I began using all the herbs and spices that flavored our meals and desserts when I was a child. Instantly, I felt more satiated with what I was eating, and didn't feel the need to gorge to get the same flavor out of food.

- Cut herbs with scissors, not knives, to prevent bruising.
- Dried herbs are more potent than fresh herbs; however, some herbs like basil and dill become relatively tasteless when dried. In general, dried herbs are best used in recipes that call for a long cooking time.
- Fresh herbs are best used in recipes when they can be added toward the end of the cooking process, since they can lose their flavor and color quickly.
- To get the most out of your herbs, rinse them thoroughly before using to make sure they're clean of dirt, sand, and any pesticides.
- To store herbs, rinse first, and then dry them completely. Wrap them in a paper towel and place them in a resealable plastic bag. They will last for at least a week. If you want, you can also place them in the freezer for up to six months. Do not freeze herbs in water, which zaps their flavor and makes them bland.
- Grinding your own spices is the best way to get the most flavor and aroma from them. Toast them lightly in the oven or in a pan over medium heat before grinding and store in a sealed container for future use.
- A clean coffee grinder is an excellent and inexpensive way to grind your own spices!
- Saffron should always be soaked for no more than 5 minutes in lukewarm water or milk, and added at the end of the dish preparation to enhance the flavor of this luxurious spice.

COOKING WITH HERBS AND SPICES

At my restaurants, we rely heavily on herbs and spices to season our food. I've noticed the American palate is a bit more sensitive, and a lighter hand is necessary when adding flavor. Too much of an aromatic can also overwhelm the subtleties in a complex recipe, ruining the dining experience.

I use a lot of dill, which many Americans see as an overwhelming herb. But the way I use it adds a subtle touch of grassy flavor to dishes like lamb stew, dolmas (stuffed grape leaves, see page 227 for recipe), and *marouli salata,* a winter salad made from romaine lettuce, scallions, and dill (see page 174 for recipe). We also use mint everywhere, for watermelon-feta salad (see page 183 for recipe) and lentil meatballs (see page 221 for recipe) to grilled vegetable soup and salmon tartare. And while most restaurants can't survive without salt and pepper, we can't live without salt, pepper, and *oregano.* This woodsy herb is in nearly every dish, but we also use it to finish plates, sprinkling oregano over almost everything that comes out of the kitchen.

I love herbs so much that I'm jealous of the signature habit of my best friend, chef Cesare Casella. He walks around with a pocket full of rosemary in his chef's coat, the scent trailing him wherever he goes. For us, there is nothing more beautiful than the natural fragrance of herbs, in the kitchen and out.

Herbs and Spices (Science)

STOP THINKING OF HERBS AND SPICES as what you *add* to food, but instead think of them as what you need *in* food to lose weight. We think herbs and spices play such an important role in fighting fat that, on the Greek Diet, we've given them their own pillar, in part to remind you that these plant-based foods should be part of your daily diet, just as they were for the ancient Greeks. Here's why herbs and spices will help you drop weight quickly, and a list of which ones to incorporate into your daily diet:

1. HERBS AND SPICES CONTAIN NATURAL CHEMICALS THAT HELP FIGHT FAT.

If it was safe, easy, and effective, would you take a drug to lose weight? Most people wouldn't think twice about saying yes. But the drug already exists—and it's called herbs and spices. These potent plant-based foods are the basis of thousands of modern pharmaceuticals that help fight colds, depression, even cancer.

Herbs and spices have potent, naturally occurring chemicals that studies show can do the following:

- Increase metabolism
- Slow gastric emptying
- Reduce blood-sugar levels
- Break up the formation of fat cells
- Decrease cravings for sugary, fatty foods

- Control appetite
- Lower the kind of inflammation that causes weight gain
- Help clear fat-storing toxins from the body

2. HERBS AND SPICES INCREASE THE FLAVOR OF FOOD WHILE REDUCING OR ELIMINATING THE NEED FOR SUGAR, SALT, AND UNHEALTHY FATS.

Most Americans rely more on sugar, salt, and unhealthy vegetable oils to flavor food, and less on herbs and spices, than people in other parts of the world. That's a huge mistake, and you don't need to be a registered dietician to figure out why: The more sugar and unhealthy oils we add to food, the greater the number of calories and effect on our blood-sugar levels.

Research also shows that sugar, salt, and unhealthy fat, especially when combined in processed foods like packaged crackers, cookies, breads, and even meat, has an effect similar to a drug, making us crave more and more of a food, even if we've eaten. Many doctors now believe these ingredients are so addictive they should be regulated just like common drugs, including alcohol and tobacco.

In comparison, adding herbs and spices to food has the opposite effect of sugar, salt, and fat, helping lower blood sugar, curtail appetite, and stop cravings cold. These seasonings have no calories, trans fats, or cholesterol, and, when used properly, flavor food with a deeper, richer, more nuanced taste than table sugar, salt, or common vegetable oil.

3. HERBS AND SPICES ADD AROMA AND COLOR TO FOOD THAT SUGAR, SALT, AND UNHEALTHY OILS CANNOT.

What sounds more filling: Chicken baked over rice . . . or chicken baked with green herbs and garlic over rice flecked by deep-red saffron and spicy black beans? Both have the same number of calories, but we're guessing the one with herbs and spices sounds tastier and more filling.

The way a food looks and smells increases our enjoyment and satiation. Herbs and spices can make the food we eat smell wonderfully rich while increasing its visual presentation, helping satisfy our noses, eyes, and stomach. On the other hand, if we flavor food only with sugar, salt, and generic vegetable oils—the standard seasonings of most home cooks and food manufacturers—

food lacks aroma and color. Increasing our use of herbs and spices is a fantastic no-calorie way to make every mouthful more enjoyable and just another part of the Mediterranean secret to losing weight.

All herbs and spices can help you lose weight for the reasons we've noted, but the following seasonings have extra-special properties to help peel off the pounds quickly:

Herb or Spice	Effect
Basil	Reduces inflammation, may help prevent aging, may help treat arthritis
Bay leaf	Reduces blood sugar levels, aids in digestion, lowers inflammation
Black pepper	Lowers blood fat levels, helps break down fat cells, helps decrease visceral (stomach) fat
Cinnamon	Lowers blood sugar, stabilizes insulin levels, delays gastric emptying
Cloves	Lowers inflammation, helps clear toxins from the body
Cumin	Reduces blood sugar levels, improves iron levels that can interfere with metabolism, aids in digestion
Dill	Reduces free radicals that cause inflammation, helps prevent unhealthy bacteria growth
Fennel	Increases metabolism, helps break down fat
Ginger	Lowers inflammation, clears toxins, increases body temperature to burn calories
Holy basil	Regulates stress hormones that cause overeating and fat storage, improves adrenal function
Horseradish	Prevents hunger pangs, lowers inflammation, helps curtail overeating
Mint	Aids in digestion, helps balance bacteria and yeast levels in the body
Oregano	May help suppress genes responsible for forming fat cells, lowers inflammation in adipose tissue
Parsley	May help the body burn fat by balancing hormone levels, acts as a natural diuretic
Red pepper, cayenne	Increases metabolism, prevents overeating, decreases cravings for sweet, salty, and fatty foods
Rosemary	Lowers inflammation, aids in digestion, increases circulation
Tumeric	Lowers inflammation, may help prevent cancer and fight infection

Fruit (Sensual)

HERE'S SOMETHING I BET most Americans have never done: Eaten a fresh fig right off the tree. It's a common occurrence in Greece, and there's nothing quite like it. I've eaten figs in other Mediterranean countries over the course of my travels, but nothing tastes like a Greek fig—sweet and juicy, crisp yet soft. I only wish everyone could taste one fig straight off the tree just once, because if they did, more people would love fruit the way I do.

We're blessed in Greece with a warm climate in which many different types of fruits can grow: oranges, clementines, apples, grapes, berries, melons, dates, plums, apricots, peaches, figs, cherries, pomegranates, pears, quince, and lemons, and that's just to name a few! In the United States, many of these fruits are imported or grown in greenhouses when they're out of season. The result is most Americans don't know the pleasure of truly fresh fruit—so much crisper, sweeter, more flavorful, and more aromatic than fruit that's transported or artificially grown. To me, fruits that aren't grown in season have no personality. In Greece, seasonality is everything—if a food isn't fresh, you don't eat it, simply because it's not available!

FRUITS IN MY YOUTH

In my village, we were lucky to be able to grow many different types of fruits, more than a dozen varieties! My favorite fruit, though, was pomegranate. This large red fruit seemed like nature's candy to me, each seed bursting with a bright, tartly flavored juice. I never craved sweets when pomegranates were in season, because I would pick one off the tree, crack it open, and eat these seeds like candy. My grandmother encouraged this by telling us pomegranates were full of antioxidants and had many health benefits, even medicinal purposes. When I was a teething toddler, for example, she would rub my gums with pomegranate seeds to numb the pain.

Of all the fruits in our village, lemons were the most widely used. My grandmother and Aunt Maria couldn't cook without them, using both the flesh and peel in many savory and sweet dishes. The juice was used for *avgolemono,* or egg-lemon sauce, a staple in Greek cooking. This is a flavorful, but healthy, dressing for so many dishes: Unlike most homemade and store-bought sauces, avgolemono doesn't have any unhealthy fats like butter and cream, but it's not packed with sugar, corn syrup, or other fattening additives, either. My grandmother used it to make chicken soup, stews, and so many other delicious dishes. (For my avgolemono recipe, see page 276.)

My family also used lemons to increase the flavor of poultry, seafood, and lamb. I learned from my grandmother that lemon juice is an excellent substitute for salt, and when combined with olive oil and fresh herbs, it makes a simple, healthy whole-food salad dressing. From my grandmother, I learned to shave lemon zest from the bitter inner rind to use to brighten heavier dishes, like lamb and tomato-based dishes; she also taught me how to use a lemon whole in syrups for desserts. My grandmother would even rub lemon juice on her hands to make them look young and soft.

We mostly ate fresh fruit, but after we harvested, we made fruit preserves, using a bit of sugar, honey, or grape must. Our homemade preserves had so much less sugar than today's commercial jams and jellies—but because they had less sugar, we had to keep them in our cellar so they wouldn't go bad. My grandmother made the best *glyka koutaliou,* or spoon desserts, with whichever fruit was in season at that time of the year: sour cherries in the spring, figs in the summer, grapes in the fall, and quince in the winter months. Today, I make a version of the dessert with cherries and honey. Make it yourself with the recipe on page 262.

ANCIENT GREEK FRUITS

The most common fruits in ancient times were olives (yes, they're a fruit!), figs, grapes, and pomegranates. The ancient Greeks would often have a fig with cheese and honey for breakfast, but more often, they ate fruit for dessert or as a snack.

Fruits held great religious significance in ancient times, specifically for the gods Zeus and

Dionysus, and the goddesses Demeter, Aphrodite, and Hera. One of their favorite dishes was an ambrosia fruit salad, made with melon, peaches, pears, grapes, and whatever fruits were in season. The ancients then dressed this healthful salad with sweet wine, honey, and nuts. The result was a delicious, healthy dessert, chock-full of fiber, vitamins, minerals, antioxidants, and protein from the nuts.

Make Your Own Ambrosia: The World's Oldest and Healthiest Dessert

To make your own ambrosia, choose different types of fresh fruit like melon, peaches, and pears. Chop the fruit into pieces so you have approximately 4 cups. Combine them in a large bowl with ½ to 1 cup grapes, and ¼ cup each chopped pistachios and almonds. In a small saucepan, simmer 1 cup sweet red wine or port with ¼ cup honey. When the mixture liquefies, pour it over the fruit and nut mixture. Chill for 1 hour before serving.

FRUITS TODAY

I always keep a green apple in my bag, because it's the perfect snack when I'm on the move. I started this habit when I was a young girl, and years later I still do it. Green apples are wonderfully crunchy, tart but sweet, and they don't bruise easily, so they're easy to pack and carry. But best of all, it's a snack that keeps me satisfied for a long time.

At my restaurants, I do my best to use local, fresh fruit to show my cooks and customers the amazing power the seasons have in determining the flavor of the food we eat. When I want a fruit that's out of season, I do what my family did—I go to the pantry. I believe in canning and preserving all the fruits from my childhood. When these fruits are at their peak, I begin the canning process. This way, I use out-of-season fruits the way we used to when I was growing up.

I enjoy using fruits in savory and sweet dishes much like my family did when I was a kid. The fruit that makes its way onto nearly every plate that leaves my kitchen is the lemon. We make the traditional Greek sauce *ladolemono,* a lemon juice and olive oil sauce that complements so many dishes, including fresh fish, simple salads, beans, and even a simple piece of bread. This sauce finishes 90 percent of my plates, adding a perfect acidity and brightness of flavor to food.

Many of my favorite desserts are made with fruit, and my top two are my homemade yogurt with spoon desserts (see page 262 for recipe), and my seasonal fresh fruit plate that uses the very best in-season fruits. It's true, some of the fruits I use now aren't native to Greece, but by sticking with the food ideology passed down through the generations, the fruit I serve is always ripe and delicious. It is better to be in tune with nature's bounty than to bend it to your will—Mother Nature's always right.

PILLAR NINE
Fruit (Science)

DESPITE WHAT SOME FAD DIETS SAY, no one ever got fat eating fruit. Quite the opposite, fruit is a key component to losing weight for a number of reasons. Studies show that people who eat more servings of fruit every day have a lower body mass index than those who don't; it's even lower than that of people who eat more vegetables. While fruit contains sugar, it's a healthier sugar than what you find in any packaged, processed food. The ancient Greeks knew it was healthy and regularly ate fruit as it's meant to be eaten, as the perfect dessert and the perfect snack—in short, Mother Nature's candy. Here are three reasons eating more fresh fruit can make you thin:

1. FRUIT FULFILLS THE URGE FOR SWEET FOODS WITHOUT CAUSING WEIGHT GAIN.

The Western world loves sugar, so much so that it's making us fat. The average American consumes six cups of sugar per week—and that's six cups of *added* sugar, not the sugar found naturally in foods (mainly fruit, dairy, and some vegetables). Think you eat a lot less sugar per week? Think again. Nearly every processed food contains added sugars, many of them hidden in foods we don't even think of as sweet. Some of the worst and most surprising offenders include packaged breads and rolls—one slice of whole wheat bread can have up to a teaspoon of sugar—salad dressings, peanut butter, tomato sauce, ketchup, and fast food. Now, add to this nearly every packaged breakfast cereal, regular fruit-sweetened yogurt, soda, and sports drink, and obvious offenders like ice cream, cake, cookies, jam, jelly, and candy, and you can see how your sugar intake can quickly top the charts.

The problem with eating too much added sugar, as most of us know, is that it causes us to gain weight—in fact, it is the number one reason for weight gain. Not only does eating foods high in added sugar drastically increase our calorie intake, doing so also causes our blood sugar to spike, triggering our bodies' production of the fat-storing hormone insulin. Increasing insulin causes us to store the calories we do eat and to make us hungrier for more sugar, fueling a vicious cycle of overeating and weight gain.

But you don't have to give up sweet foods altogether—in fact, research shows that including a little sugar in your diet can help you lose weight. Fruit contains sugar, but it's not an added sugar; it's a natural sugar called fructose. Do not confuse this with high-fructose corn syrup, a highly refined type of fructose found in many packaged foods that studies show increases cravings and causes our bodies to store more fat. By comparison, the natural fructose found in fruit does not cause fat storage or weight gain. Quite the opposite: A recent study published in the journal *Metabolism* found that people lost significantly more weight eating a diet that contained fruit with natural fructose than eating a low-fructose diet.

The best way to use fruit to lose weight is to eat it whenever you want something sweet, whether that's over your cereal or yogurt in the morning, sliced into your salad at lunch, during the day as a snack, or after dinner as a dessert. The more fruit you eat as a substitute for higher-calorie foods, the more weight you'll lose.

Swap High-Calorie Snacks for Fruit

Instead of:	Eat:
Sugar on cereal, yogurt, and oatmeal	Berries, sliced mangoes, peaches, or pomegranate seeds
Cookies and crackers	Crunchy fruit like apples or pears
Candy	Regular or frozen grapes
Cake and pie	Fruit salad, baked apples, or pears with honey
Soda	Seltzer water with lemon, lime, or orange slices
Croutons on salad	Sliced pears, berries, or pomegranate seeds
Chips	Baked Apple Chips (page 279)

2. FRUIT CONTAINS A DOUBLE WHAMMY OF FIBER AND WATER TO HELP CURB HUNGER AND TRIGGER WEIGHT LOSS.

Just like vegetables and beans, fruit is a fantastic source of the kind of natural fibers shown to make us feel full while lowering our blood-sugar levels and helping clear fat-storing toxins from the body. Like vegetables and beans, fruit also contains both natural insoluble and soluble fibers, the combination science has found most effective for increasing satiety, slowing gastric emptying, and causing weight loss (see Pillar Four: Beans for more details on how these natural fibers help our bodies fight fat).

Here are the fruits highest in fiber to help fill you up and trigger fiber's fat-burning effects:

HIGH-FIBER FRUITS

FRUIT	FIBER (G)
Raspberries, 1 cup	8
Blackberries, 1 cup	7.6
Pomegranate seeds, 1 cup	6
Pear, 1 medium	5.6
Apple, 1 medium	4.4
Blueberries, 1 cup	3.6
Banana, 1 medium	3.1

Fruit also contains a lot of water, helping prevent dehydration, which interferes with weight loss, while increasing the volume of food to help fill us up. But that's not all. As we learned in Pillar Three: Vegetables, when fiber is combined with water in a food, it provides a double whammy for weight loss. Water helps soluble fiber expand in our stomachs, forming a viscous gel that reduces hunger and makes us feel as if we've eaten more than we have. Finally, the more water in a food, the fewer calories it has by volume. Vegetables have the highest water content of any food, averaging about 90 percent, but whole fruit trails closely, with most types of fruit having a water content ranging between 80 and 90 percent.

Eating more whole, fresh fruit will help you lose weight, but eating dried fruit and fruit juice can have the opposite effect. While they contain some of the micronutrients found in fruit, dried fruit and juice are high in sugar and calories by volume, and juice lacks fruit's fat-burning fiber and can contain added sugars. For these reasons, steer clear of juice altogether, and apply the Greeks' favorite motto—*metron ariston,* "everything in moderation"—when eating dried fruit, using it in small amounts in everyday dishes like salad and yogurt.

3. FRUIT IS RICH IN MICRONUTRIENTS THAT BOOST METABOLISM AND BURN FAT.

We've all heard the saying "An apple a day keeps the doctor away." And there's a reason why that motto has stuck as a popular maxim. Fruit is packed with the vitamins, minerals, and antioxidants that research shows can help prevent a number of chronic illnesses, from heart disease, diabetes, and cancer to osteoporosis, Parkinson's, Alzheimer's, asthma, arthritis, and colds and flu.

These same micronutrients also help fight what's quickly becoming the most widespread disease in the Western world: obesity. The vitamins, minerals, and antioxidants found in fruit help every system in our bodies function on a higher level, including our bodies' metabolism. Studies show the common micronutrients found naturally in fruit, like potassium, folate, and vitamin C, increase our bodies' metabolic rate, allowing us to burn more calories at rest. What's more, these micronutrients also help give us more energy to move more throughout our day and exercise. Finally, antioxidants and other natural compounds found in fruit not only prevent premature aging (which is why fruit is a common ingredient in top-of-the-line antiaging skin care products), they also work overtime to fight the free radicals that interfere with optimal metabolism and digestion.

Coffee and Tea (Sensual)

THE FIRST THING I DO every morning is have a cup of Greek coffee, along with a glass of water. This isn't like any American coffee you've had—it's rich and thickly flavored, an unstrained coffee made from finely ground beans and served in a demitasse. I keep adding water to my cup, little by little, to make the coffee last for several hours. This is my morning ritual, drinking the coffee while I prepare for the day, reading emails, checking on kitchen orders, scheduling meetings, and working on recipes. The coffee gives me a gentle, warming energy that helps wake me up while also relaxing me—when I have my morning cup of coffee, it is my time to think and embrace the day.

The same way I start the day, I end it—not with a cup of Greek coffee, but with a mug of traditional Greek tea called mountain tea. Every night when I get home, I brew a fresh pot of tea on the stove. Like Greek coffee, mountain tea gives me a gentle, warming feeling, too, which helps settle me for the day and relax me before bed. I find the ritual of these two drinks part of a healthy balanced life, and as I learned from my people, coffee and tea are two of the healthiest beverages you can drink.

GROWING UP WITH COFFEE AND TEA

I always loved the smell of freshly brewed Greek coffee as a child. When I was five years old, my grandmother taught me how to make the brew for my grandfather so I could impress him. (To see how we brew Greek coffee, turn to page 283.) He told me if I did a good job making his coffee, he would take me to the *kafeneo*, the coffee shop where all the men in the village would gather in the afternoons to talk about the past, the future, and everything in between.

It wasn't until I was seven that I first tasted Greek coffee. My grandfather let me sip from his cup, but warned me not to drink it again until I was older because it wasn't good for kids. He said it would make me nervous because I was already full of energy, and it was true. But when I grew older, this was no longer the case—the energy from Greek coffee was steady and consistent, not abrupt with the sudden, subsequent crash of some American blends that contain more caffeine.

Mountain tea, on the other hand, I had all the time as a child. This tea is made from dried herbs of the plant *sideritis* and usually served with honey and lemon. My mother would make it for my siblings and me before we went to bed to calm us from the day and lull us to sleep. In the winter months, she would make us chicken soup for dinner and mountain tea before bed to ensure we awoke feeling good and healthy. Anytime I wasn't feeling well, I would drink this tea because everyone in my village knew it could help treat many sicknesses, from colds and flus to digestive problems and sleep disorders. As I got older, I drank mountain tea more and more, every few hours throughout the day. It was like a cleansing tonic, helping to make my mind sharper and my body stronger.

TEA IN ANCIENT GREECE

Although coffee was not found in ancient Greece, mountain tea was a popular drink among all classes of people. Even the poor could harvest the wild herb in the mountains, and they would brew the tea over their fires during the day and at night. They used the tea as a digestive aid and to help cure colds and other illnesses.

Sideritis translates literally as "he who is or has the iron." The ancient Greeks gave the herb this name because sideritis was well known to have properties capable of healing soldiers' wounds caused by iron weapons during battle. It turns out the ancient Greeks knew something about the plant that took scientists years to figure out: Sideritis is high in iron, which is why, in some countries, it's also called ironwort.

COFFEE AND TEA TODAY

When I began my career as a lobbyist, I started drinking coffee like the Italians do: with milk and sugar. I enjoyed the flavor and aroma of the beans very much, but didn't like stirring in the fattening additions my contemporaries seemed to thrive on.

Several years later, my good Greek friend Eva Zach asked me, "You speak about Greece all over the world, and you don't drink the best thing to come out of your country?" I was visiting her home in Greece, and she had just made me a cup of Greek coffee, something I hadn't had in years. I was instantly taken back to my childhood and blown away by the intense flavor and unique texture of the beverage that some refer to as "the sludge." Right then and there, I vowed to start drinking Greek coffee again, and I've never stopped. What's so great about the beverage is that you don't need to add sugar or milk—and most Greeks drink it without either!

Unfortunately, I also stopped drinking my traditional mountain tea when I was eating like a Westerner. But when I changed back to a traditional Greek diet, I started drinking the tea again. I remember visiting the sea near my home village, and sitting on the beach with my cup of hot mountain tea, with my feet in the ocean. It was so relaxing—the hot tea and cold ocean—and I thought to myself, "Why did I ever stop drinking mountain tea?" I felt stronger instantly, even more eager to commit to my new healthier way of eating.

As a chef in New York City, I feel it is important to offer a selection of coffees and teas that my diners are familiar and comfortable with. However, I always encourage patrons to try the Greek coffee and the mountain tea—and the result is often that they become committed Greek coffee or tea drinkers who order it every time they come in. If one of my friends isn't feeling well, I always send a package of mountain tea, with a jar of honey and some fresh lemons, and instructions on how to properly brew the tea. (See the recipe for Greek Mountain Tea on page 284.) The harsh winters in New York are the perfect setting to finish a delicious Greek meal with a hot cup of Greek coffee or mountain tea.

Although some cultures cook with coffee and tea, this style of cuisine is not native to the Mediterranean. Greeks don't cook with these beverages—we prefer to drink them instead. There is no better way to start your day or to end it than with a cup of a warm, filling drink. Like wine, I strongly believe that no meal is complete without a cup of hot coffee or tea.

PILLAR TEN

Coffee and Tea (Science)

FORGET EVERYTHING you've ever heard about coffee—most of it is inaccurate. While the ancient Greek motto *metron ariston* (everything in moderation) holds true here, science shows drinking coffee, along with tea, can not only boost your health and longevity, but doing so is also an important tool to help you lose weight.

The ancient Greeks (and Maria!) enjoyed a type of boiled coffee known as Greek coffee, which studies show is high in heart-healthy compounds. But you can still get the same weight-loss effects from a standard cup of joe. Similarly, Maria likes traditional Greek mountain tea, but you can get the same effect from many different types of tea. Here's everything you need to know about losing weight on nature's no-calorie fat-burning brews of champions:

> If you have a serious medical condition or trouble sleeping, check with your doctor before increasing your intake of caffeinated drinks.

1. CAFFEINATED COFFEE AND TEA INCREASE METABOLISM AND HELP REGULATE FAT-STORING INSULIN.

Trials with caffeinated coffee and tea show that drinking a cup of either increases metabolism significantly by stimulating the central nervous system. In fact, a study published in the journal *Physiology & Behavior* found that drinking 1 cup of regular coffee can boost your metabolic rate by as much as 16 percent compared to drinking decaf coffee—or no coffee at all! The natural caffeine found in tea has the same effect, but research shows certain compounds in green and oolong teas may elevate metabolism more than black or white teas.

However, caffeinated coffees and teas do more than add an instant rev to our caloric burn as we go about our days. Research shows that people who regularly drink coffee regulate blood sugar and insulin more effectively, preventing fat storage as well as lowering the risk of diabetes. However, remember the ancient Greek motto, *metron ariston* (everything in moderation): Studies show that drinking more than 5 cups of regular American coffee a day (the equivalent of 10 cups of Greek coffee or 10 cups of caffeinated tea) can have the opposite effect, increasing glucose intolerance.

Greek Coffee: The Secret to Long Life

Scientists know coffee is good for us, but recent research shows boiled Greek coffee beats all other brews when it comes to boosting our hearts and overall health. One study of nearly 700 people on the Greek island of Ikaria, which has one of the highest longevity rates in the world, found that drinking the traditional coffee helped improve cardiovascular function in older people, even those with blood pressure problems. Researchers credit the effect to the fact that Greek coffee is higher in certain heart-healthy antioxidant compounds and lower in caffeine than regular filtered coffee, providing a more consistent energy surge.

2. CAFFEINATED COFFEE AND TEA BOOST YOUR MOTIVATION TO WORK OUT—AND THE NUMBER OF CALORIES YOU BURN WHEN YOU DO.

Tired or just can't motivate to get outside for the walk or jog you know will make you feel better and more energetic? Drink a cup of coffee or nonherbal tea to help you get on your way. These are such powerful antidotes to preworkout lethargy that most professional athletes wouldn't think about undertaking a workout without a little help from Mother Nature, despite the fact they're essentially getting paid to exercise. While most of us don't have a paycheck dangling at the end of a brisk walk, run, bike, dance, or trip to the gym, we can use the next best thing.

The natural caffeine found in regular coffee and nonherbal tea increases energy in a number of ways. First, caffeine breaks down fat cells, liberating fatty acids inside, which then enter our bloodstream and provide a surge of energy. Second, studies show caffeine helps improve focus, alertness, and concentration, boosting the motivation you may need not only to pull those classic all-nighters in college, but also to follow through on a workout regimen. Similarly, caffeine helps improve our mood, lifting the fog of irritability or sadness that sometimes prevents us from moving our bodies like they were made to move.

Once we start exercising, the effects of drinking caffeinated coffee or tea start working overtime to help our bodies burn more fat. It's no secret that caffeine enhances exercise performance, helping us work out harder and longer, ultimately allowing our bodies to burn more calories. But caffeinated drinks do more than that: Research from the Australian Institute of Sport shows that consuming caffeine before exercise helps the muscles burn fat for fuel instead of carbs, tapping into actual fat cells rather than firing off circulating blood glucose. Finally, caffeine helps reduce muscle pain when we work out, making us enjoy the experience that much more—and entices us to want to repeat it that much more often.

The Problem with Energy Drinks

While we highly encourage drinking caffeinated coffee and tea on the Greek Diet, we strongly discourage caffeinated energy drinks like Red Bull, Monster, and even those marketed as being natural, like Organic Energy. Not only are these concoctions loaded with sugar, calories, and harmful chemicals, they also contain synthetic caffeine, often in concentrated forms, all of which research has shown produces a jolt in energy and a subsequent crash. Studies have also found energy drinks can have dangerous effects on heart rate, blood pressure, and brain function, largely due to a combination of concentrated synthetic caffeine and other stimulants.

---

3. COFFEE AND TEA INCREASE FEELINGS OF FULLNESS, REDUCE APPETITE, AND HELP PREVENT CRAVINGS AND OVEREATING.

Have you ever had a cup of coffee or tea in the morning and subsequently lost all interest in eating breakfast? It's not just you: Studies show that the caffeine in coffee or strong nonherbal teas like black and oolong can help curb appetite and increase feelings of fullness. The effect is so strong the National Institutes of Health warns those who don't want to lose weight, like children, that drinking too much caffeine will suppress appetite to the point of weight loss.

But coffee—and tea to some extent—has an effect on our hunger and feelings of fullness that goes beyond caffeine. A recent study published in the *Journal of the American College of Nutrition* found a compound in decaffeinated coffee that decreases hunger and increases our bodies' satiety hormone, PPY. Similarly, research from *Nutrition Journal* shows drinking green tea can significantly boost feelings of fullness, both when consumed on its own and after a meal.

Many people also find that a warm cup of coffee or tea, taken with a little milk and even sugar or honey, can help satisfy an urge for something sweet or savory after a meal and even prevent overeating. Just be sure to use milk instead of cream to keep your saturated fat intake in check and be careful with how much sugar you put in your coffee or tea—and remember that artificial sweeteners like Splenda and Equal have been shown to cause weight gain, among other health problems. A no-calorie fat-burning drink can quickly turn into a fattening high-calorie dessert if you add enough milk or cream, along with sugar.

WHEN COFFEE BECOMES WORSE THAN CAKE

Drinking coffee and tea on the Greek Diet will help you lose weight. But drinking coffee or tea drinks—lattes, frappes, mochas, cappuccinos, and chais—will cause you to gain weight. These specialty drinks are packed with so much sugar and so many calories that coffee and tea's fat-burning properties are quickly negated. Just how bad are coffee and tea drinks for your waistline? A venti white chocolate mocha from Starbucks, for example, has 580 calories—30 more than a McDonald's Big Mac—and a whopping 75 grams of sugar, which is nearly three times the amount found in a regular-size Snickers bar. Tea drinks are no better: A venti green tea latte from Starbucks has 450 calories and 71 grams of sugar!

---

4. COFFEE AND TEA ARE AN EASY NO-CALORIE WAY TO ADD MORE METABOLISM-BOOSTING ANTIOXIDANTS TO YOUR DIET.

Here's a fun bit of trivia for your next watercooler moment: Coffee is America's number one source of antioxidants. While this in part means most Americans aren't eating enough of the antioxidant-rich plants central to the Greek Diet, it also goes to show you how many healthy plant compounds are in one of the world's oldest and most cherished beverages. In part for this reason, coffee has been shown by research to increase longevity and protect against cognitive decline and diseases like Parkinson's. Studies have also found that those who drink coffee regularly have lower rates of many types of cancer.

Not to be overlooked, black, green, white, and oolong teas are also high in different types of antioxidants, and drinking both coffee and tea daily can help boost your intake of these healthy plant compounds considerably. Just be sure to watch your overall daily caffeine intake, and don't shun decaf: Decaf coffee and regular tea (not herbal) are also rich in antioxidants and contain many of the compounds that can help your body burn fat.

Health Benefits of Greek Mountain Tea

Greek mountain tea has been used for centuries as a powerful medicinal for nearly every ailment, including digestive problems, colds and flu, asthma, even pain. Today, studies show the traditional drink, made from the dried leaves and flowers of the ironwort (*sideritis*) plant, is an effective anti-inflammatory and antimicrobial, helping relieve upper respiratory symptoms, allergies, and other illnesses. In addition, Greek mountain tea contains certain antioxidants research suggests may help prevent cancer. You can find the tea online and at gourmet food and tea shops.

Nuts and Seeds (Sensual)

NO GREEK KITCHEN IS COMPLETE without nuts and seeds, especially walnuts, almonds, sesame seeds, pistachios, and pine nuts. At my restaurants, nuts make their way into at least half of my menu items. Often patrons ask why they appear so frequently, and my response comes from my chef mentality—texture and flavor, I tell them. But I also know nuts and seeds add a healthy crunch to nearly every dish, savory and sweet.

My love of nuts began in the mountain ranges surrounding my village, where walnut trees grew wild. We would go as a family up into the mountains to harvest the nuts, shaking them straight off the trees. We would lay blankets below the trunks, so we could quickly bundle up our bounty. We would also pick the walnuts directly off the lower branches, our hands turning black with the oil from the shells, as we added even more nuts to our bundles. We would then tie our blankets onto the end of a stick, and walk back to our village like hobos, our big bags of walnuts swinging behind us. But we didn't feel like hobos—we felt like we were on top of the world with our bags of goodies, knowing all the delicious treats we could make and that the nuts we carried would keep us wise, happy, and healthy for the rest of the year.

GROWING UP A NUT

When I was a child, my father told my sisters, brother, and me that if we wanted to be clever, we had to eat a handful of almonds and walnuts every morning. I was perfectly happy to eat my dose fresh out of my family's pantry, but my preference was to sprinkle my daily handful on top of some of my mother's fresh yogurt.

My grandmother was "the ruler of the nuthouse," as my grandfather called her. She loved nuts and taught us how to harvest walnuts from the mountains. She also taught us how to sort through the nuts to find the bad ones, shaking them to make sure they were full and plump, and my siblings and I worked like an assembly line doing just that to make sure we kept only the best walnuts. (I still sort out bad walnuts in my kitchen—if a walnut shell doesn't make any noise when you shake it, it's bad.)

My grandmother used the walnuts we sorted to bake her famous baklava, a nut dessert made with phyllo dough and honey. I was the lucky one who got to help her, grinding the nuts and beating the olive oil into a froth that she used to coat the phyllo dough. I can still smell the rich aroma of roasted walnuts from her baklava baking in the oven. Today, I make my own version of my grandmother's recipe, but have made it far healthier and tastier than most Americanized or traditional versions. (For my baklava recipe, see page 257.)

Another of my childhood favorites is now a popular American snack—peanut butter. But unlike in most homes in the United States today, we made our own peanut butter. My grandmother used a mortar and pestle to hand-grind a pound of peanuts, adding two tablespoons of olive oil and a pinch of salt for a creamy blend. Unlike commercial peanut butters today, she didn't add any sugar, preservatives, or other additives. The result was a healthy, thick spread high in protein and rich in healthy fats. My grandmother would give it to us as a snack after school, before we did our homework, telling us it would make us strong and smart.

Twice a year, my father would travel to the northern city of Thessaloniki, always returning with two large tins of Haitoglou sesame oil, a native brand of oil in Greece. This is absolutely the best sesame oil you can find, even today, because the company, Haitoglou, only makes it from scratch, using the high-quality sesame seeds grown on its farm. (You can order this from Greece—visit the Haitoglou website at www.sesame.gr/en/haitoglou.htm.) In this oil, Aunt Maria would often pan-fry fish, vegetables, and her homemade meatballs. She also baked bread with sesame seeds and made a delicious dessert from sesame seeds and honey called *sisamopites* that all the children in my neighborhood would ask for—this was our Greek version of candy.

The Trick to Toasting Nuts

Put a skillet over high heat until the pan is very hot. Turn the flame to low and add the nuts. Constantly stir and redistribute the nuts until you can smell the nuts' aroma. When this happens, remove them from the pan. Do not overcook or they will become bitter.

NUTS AND SEEDS IN ANCIENT GREECE

Many of the nuts and seeds we use today were consumed in abundance in ancient Greece, including almonds, chestnuts, peanuts, pistachios, walnuts, and sesame seeds. The ancients ate nuts as a snack and added them to many meals. They believed eating nuts would help increase personal wisdom and overall health.

The ancient Greeks used sesame seeds to develop the world's first energy bar, a popular snack called *pasteli* that was considered to be food for warriors. The Greeks made pasteli by mixing sesame seeds and honey into a flat cake, like Aunt Maria did, then baking the cake until it hardened. This was an easy snack for warriors to pack and eat in battle camps or when traveling. The ancients believed pasteli would give their warriors extra strength and pleasure, helping them fight longer and harder.

Walnuts are arguably one of the most Greek of ingredients, in part because the ancients are credited with first cultivating the nut. The Greeks called walnuts the "royal nut" and grew them in abundance in fields. When Zeus, the father of all Olympian gods, would spend time on Earth, he would feast on walnuts for additional strength and wisdom. Similarly, the ancients believed walnuts had specific medicinal purposes, capable even of counteracting strong poisons when combined with figs and roux (flour and water).

I'VE GONE NUTS!

Even during my dark days eating as a Westerner, I never gave up nuts. When I was traveling, I always tried to find nuts produced in Greece, especially pistachios from Aegina, an island off the coast of Athens. Aegina pistachios were so flavorful and tasty because the seawater produces a better nut, satisfying in a way processed snacks never are. After a long day at work, I would unwind with a glass of red wine and some pistachios, enjoying the feeling of breaking open the shell to find the green nut inside.

I still eat nuts every day, keeping little bowls of nuts around the house, and whenever I'm hungry and too busy to sit down for yogurt, I scoop a little handful for myself. Of course, nuts are in most meals I make for myself and for my patrons. When it comes to nuts, I'm literally nuts about them! Nuts are the perfect multipurpose ingredient: I use them to help bind soups; to add texture to sauces; to garnish salads, pastas, and seafood dishes; and to fill desserts like baklava and parfaits. For just about every culinary application I can think of, there is a nut to use. I grind walnuts to use as a crust for chicken and meats, and I even make my own Greek stuffing for Thanksgiving out of chestnuts, almonds, walnuts, and pine nuts.

I also like to cook with nut and seed oils, particularly cold-pressed sesame oil, which, in my opinion, is second only to olive oil! In moderation, this cost-effective oil is a must and luxurious way to flavor foods like fish, root vegetables, and squashes. With a high smoke point, it adds a wonderful golden color and texture to foods.

Sesame paste, or tahini, is also extremely useful in the traditional Mediterranean kitchen. This creamy paste is a cornerstone of Greek cooking, used in signature dishes like hummus (see page 270 for recipe), *tahinosoupa* (tahini vegetable soup, page 189), and *halva*, a nut-honey dessert. Tahini can also help you shave calories and unhealthy fat by acting as a great substitute for butter and jam on bread. You can also swap it for eggs in many sauces, a perfect trick when cooking or baking vegan meals.

Make Your Own Nut Butter in Five Minutes

Choose whichever nut you want for your butter: peanuts, cashews, almonds, and/or walnuts. If you want, toast them for 30 seconds in a hot pan over low heat—this helps bring out a nut's natural essence. Add the nuts to a food processor and process on high. When you see the mixture begin to form a ball, slowly drizzle in a tablespoon or two of extra-virgin olive oil (or the oil of the nut you're using) and salt, if desired, while continuing to process. Process until you are happy with the texture. Store your butter in an airtight container in the refrigerator (to extend shelf life, as we don't use preservatives!).

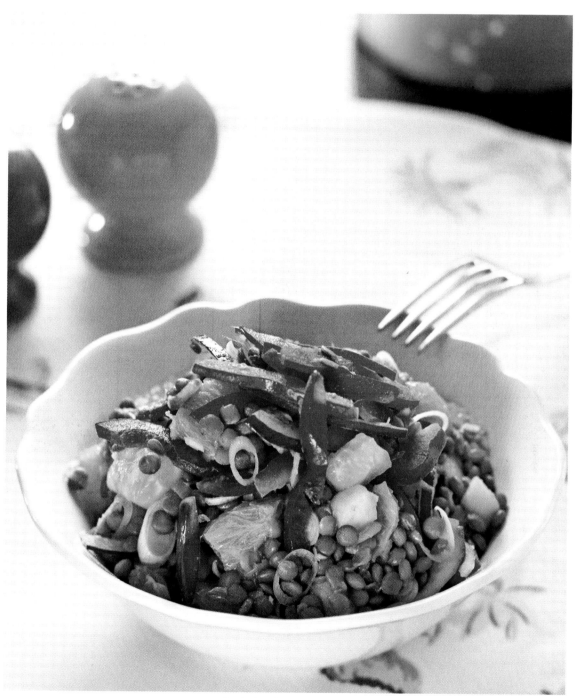

Lentil Salad with Oranges, page 176

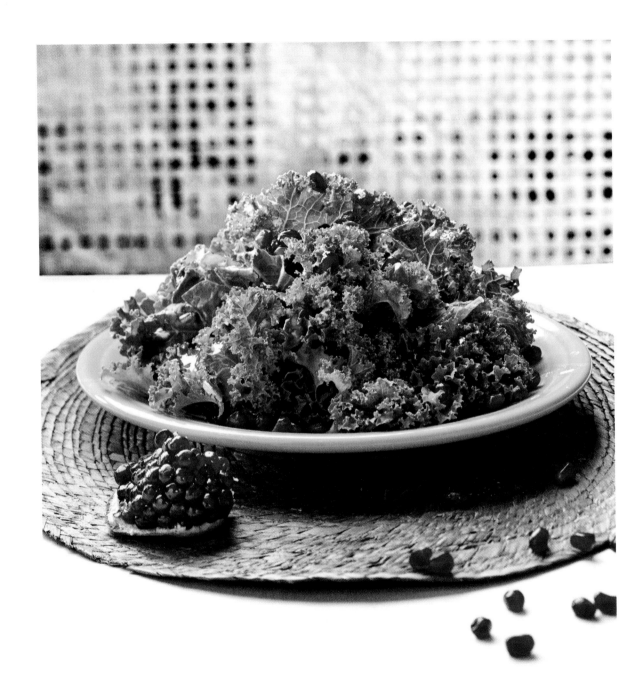

Pomegranate-Kale Salad, page 178

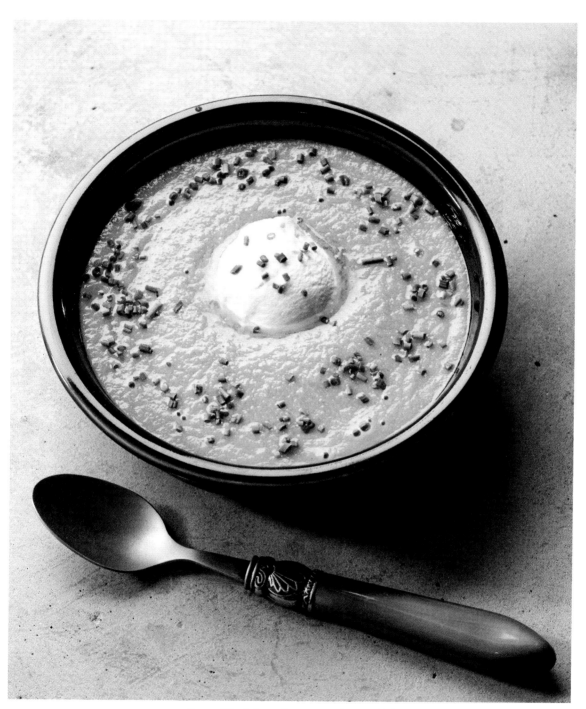

Pea and Leek Soup (Hortosoupa), page 185

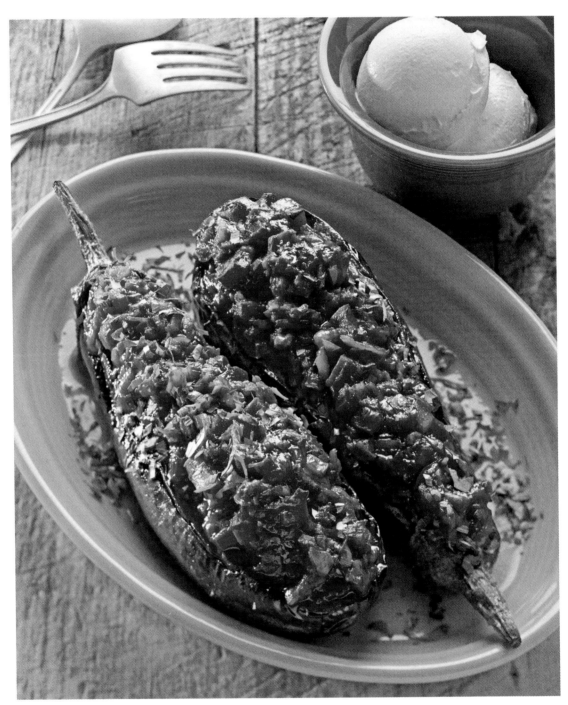

Stuffed Baby Eggplant (Papoutsakia), page 198

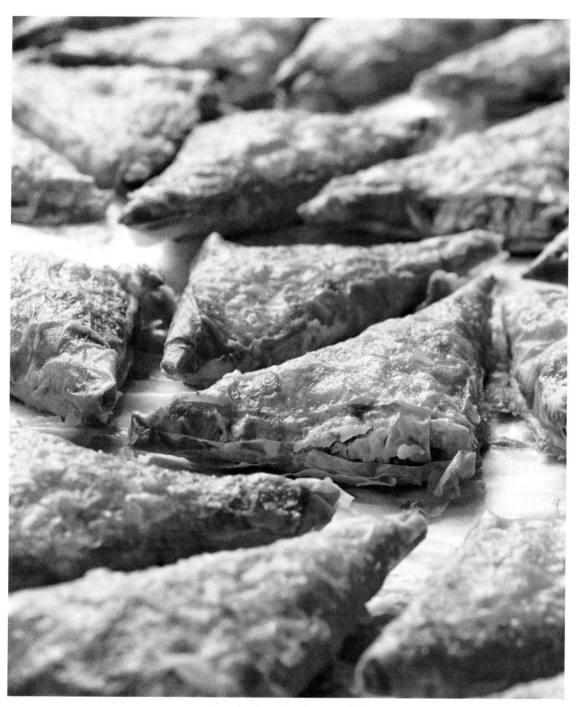

Spanakopita Triangles, page 206

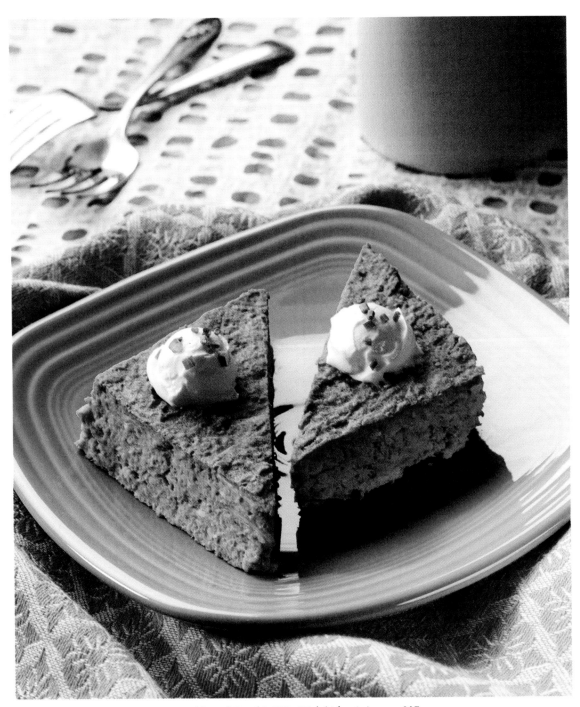
Pumpkin and Zucchini Pie (Kolokithopita), page 207

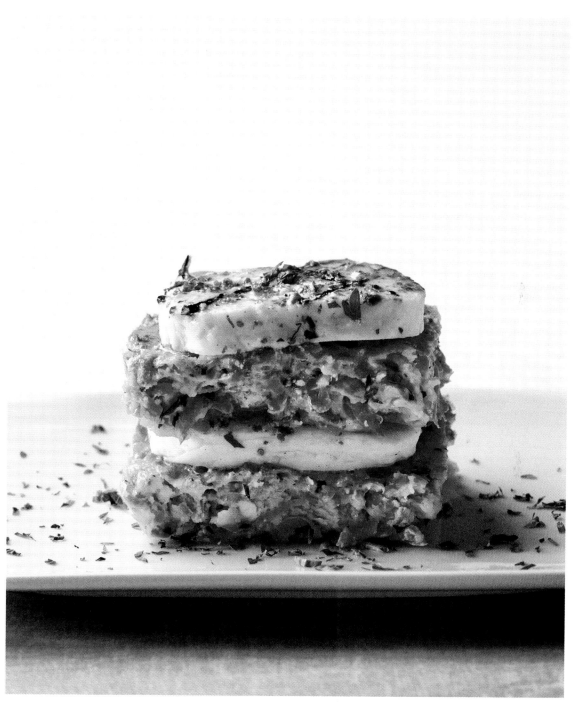

Carrot and Halloumi Croquettes (Karotopites Me Halloumi), page 210

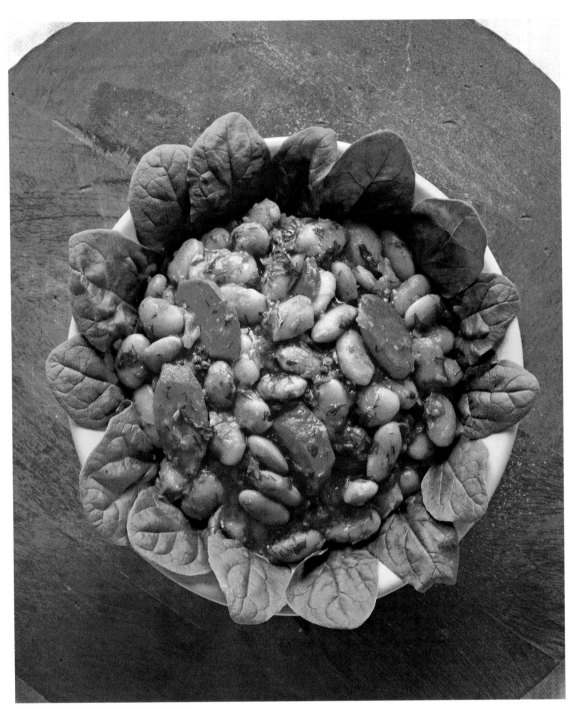

Braised Giant Beans with Spinach (Gigantes Me Spanaki), page 218

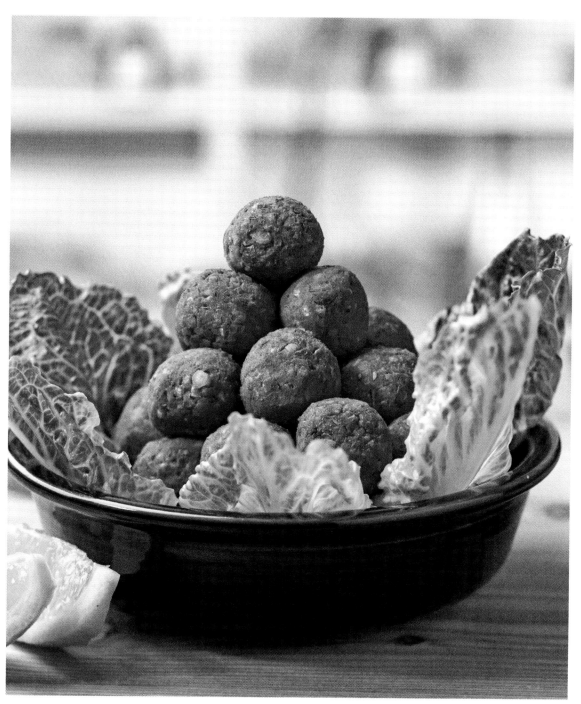

Cold Red Lentil Faux Meatballs, page 221

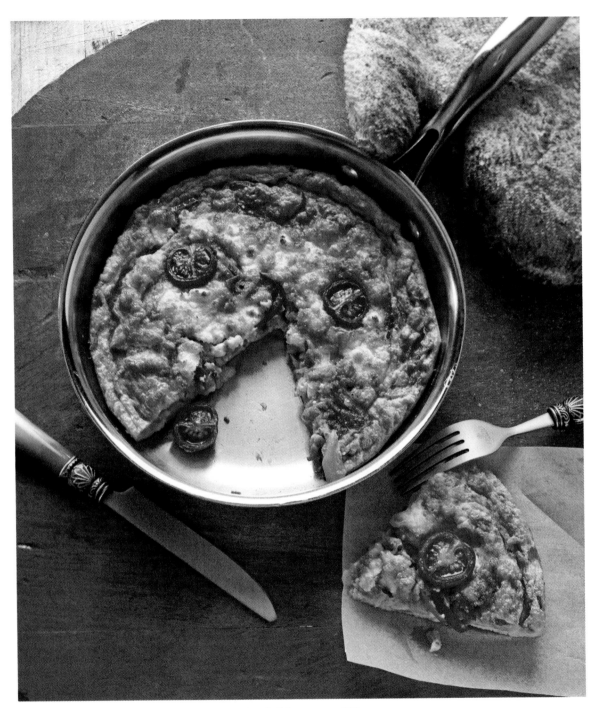

Greek Frittata, page 225

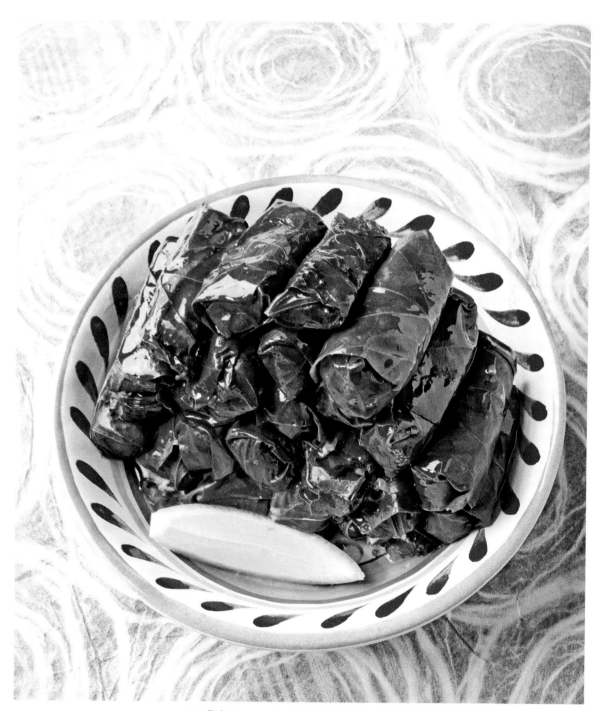

Stuffed Grape Leaves (Dolmadakia), page 227

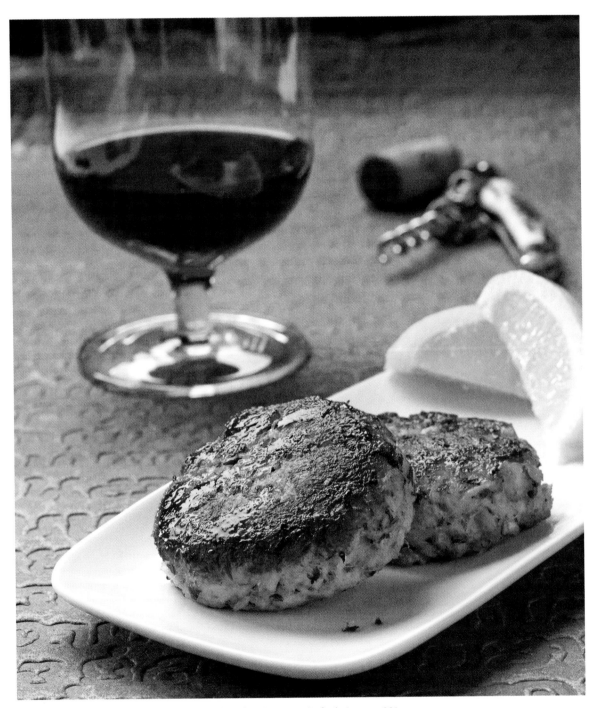
Crab Cakes (Kavourokeftedes), page 231

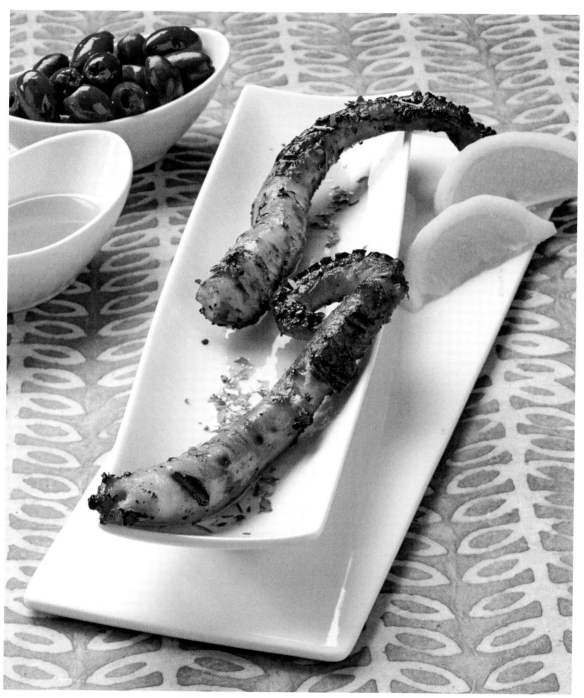

Grilled Octopus (Htapodaki Stin Schara), page 236

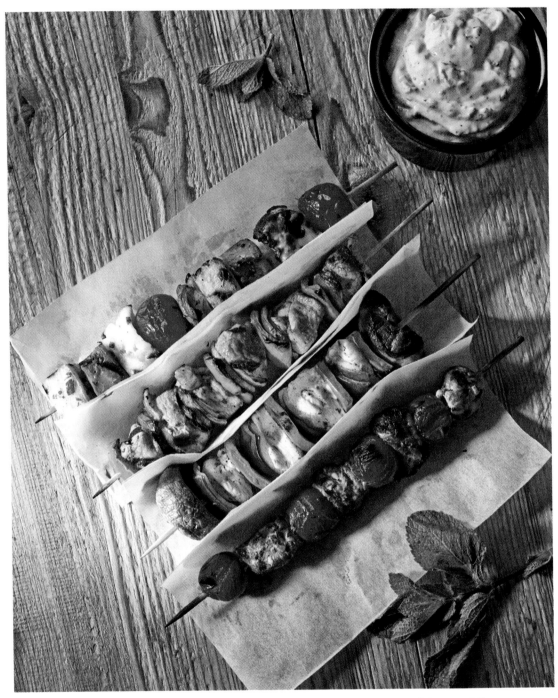

Souvlaki *(from top to bottom)*: Vegetable Souvlaki, page 192; Lamb Souvlaki, page 245; Chicken and Mushroom Souvlaki, page 254; Salmon Souvlaki, page 239

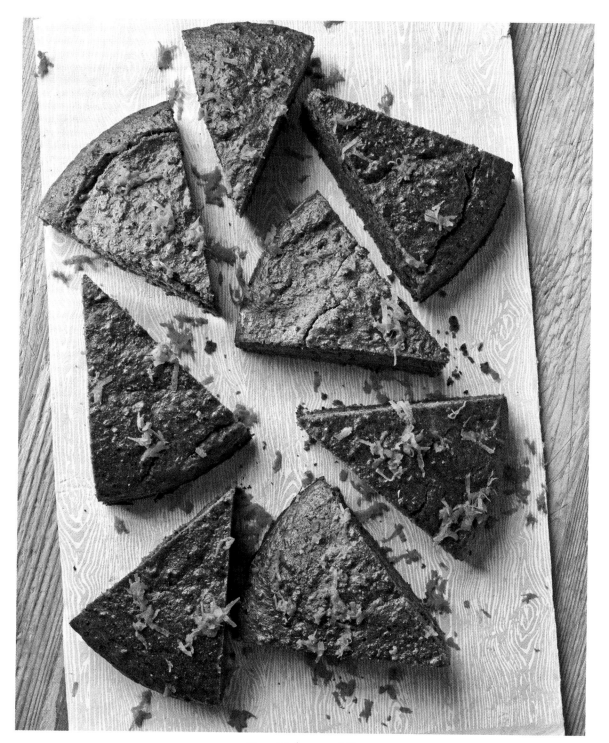

Carrot Cake, page 266

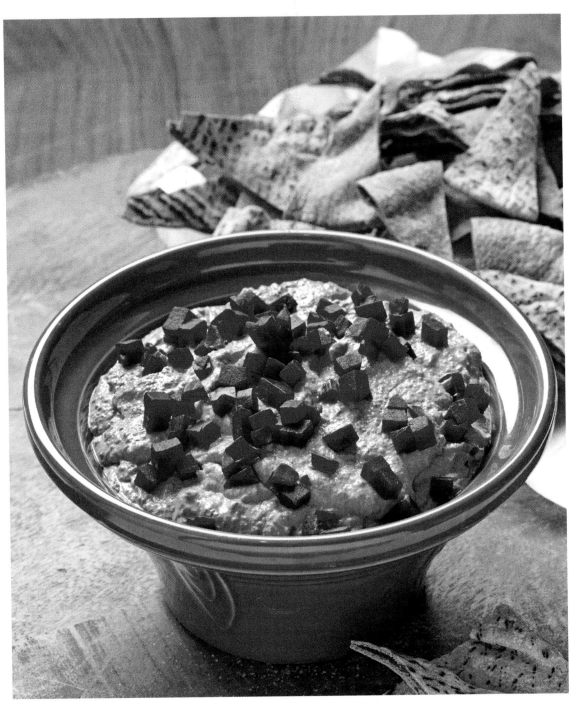

Roasted Beet–Yogurt Dip, page 275

Nuts and Seeds (Science)

CRUNCHY, RICH, FLAVORFUL, FATTY, and sometimes salty. Sound like a diet food? It is. We're talking about nuts. They are nature's healthiest snack, whether you're trying to lose weight, maintain your current weight, lower your cholesterol, and prevent heart disease and even cancer, according to new research. Sure, nuts—and seeds—are high in fat and calories, but science shows consuming the type of fat found in them in moderation helps us curb cravings, increase satiety, and even burn body fat.

We feel so strongly about nuts and seeds, in fact, that we believe if everyone swapped a handful of nuts for processed snacks like potato chips, corn chips, crackers, and cookies, most of us would drop five pounds in a month's time without making any other dietary changes. Sounds too easy, right? It is.

We also believe, like the ancient Greeks did, that adding nuts and seeds to desserts, sauces, salads, and entrées can make them so filling, you simply will not be able to overeat—a superb trick if you have a tendency toward night or binge eating, or just never feel full after meals. Here's why we recommend you eat a handful of nuts or seeds (1.5 ounces) as a snack or as part of your meals every day:

1. NUTS AND SEEDS CONTAIN HIGH AMOUNTS OF NEARLY EVERY NUTRIENT SHOWN TO BOOST METABOLISM, LOWER BLOOD SUGAR, AND BURN FAT.

If there's a nutrient science suggests can help improve a sluggish metabolism and prevent fat storage, it's most likely found in nuts and some seeds. These tiny little powerhouses are packed with the major macronutrients we already know help fill us up and curtail hunger: protein, fiber, and healthy fat. But nuts and seeds also contain dozens of micronutrients like magnesium and vitamin E that have specific—and significant—fat-burning advantages. Here's the skinny on what you're getting in a handful of nuts:

- **Fat:** Nuts on average are made up of 80 percent fat by weight; most seeds are just slightly lower in fat. The fat in nuts and seeds is largely monounsaturated, or MUFA, which is also found in olive oil. As we learned in Pillar One: Olive Oil, MUFA increases fat oxidization, or our bodies' ability to use fat as a fuel source. Studies have also found that eating more MUFA instead of the saturated fat found in most snacks increases your resting energy expenditure. In addition, nuts contain a type of MUFA known as oleic acid, which is also present in olive oil and which studies show increases our bodies' production of hunger-curbing hormones. Finally, nuts and seeds contain plant-based omega-3 fatty acids. While not as beneficial to weight loss as the marine-based fatty acids found in fish, plant-based omega-3s help right our bodies' critical balance between inflammation-causing omega-6 fats and inflammation-lowering omega-3s.

- **Fiber:** A handful of nuts or seeds has around 5 grams of fiber—not bad for a snack on the go, especially when you consider the same serving size of potato chips or cookies has zero stomach-satiating fiber. Most nuts contain naturally occurring soluble and insoluble fiber, the combination that can help speed weight loss more than synthetic fibers or strictly insoluble fiber.

- **Protein:** Enjoy a 1.5-ounce serving of almonds (about 30 almonds) and you'll get 9 grams of hunger-stopping protein. When you compare the protein in nuts to that of most snack foods, with the exception of Greek yogurt, you'll find nuts are an ideal choice to keep your protein intake high and processed carb count low.

- **Magnesium:** A handful of nuts packs almost 60 percent of our recommended daily allowance for magnesium—more than what's in a cup of spinach! This mineral is critical to a healthy metabolism—and it's also sorely lacking in the Western diet, with Americans consuming on average only 66 percent of the needed daily amount of magnesium. Without an abundance of this mineral, our bodies cannot properly digest, absorb, and use the protein, fat, and carbs we eat. Groundbreaking research also suggests a high magnesium intake can even prevent obesity genes from expressing themselves.

• **Vitamin E:** One serving of almonds (1.5 ounces) contains more than 50 percent of your recommended daily vitamin E intake. Why care about this fat-soluble vitamin? Not only do 90 percent of Americans fall short in their recommended daily allowance, studies show nutritional vitamin E found in foods can help boost immune health, prevent cognitive disease, improve skin moisture and appearance, and may stop plaque from forming along artery walls. Better yet, vitamin E also helps us lose weight. Strong research suggests vitamin E helps improve insulin resistance, thereby preventing our bodies from holding on to fat.

• **Manganese:** A handful of the Greeks' beloved pine nuts provides a whopping 180 percent of your recommended daily allowance for the trace mineral manganese. This overlooked micronutrient's primary function is activating enzymes in the body that help to facilitate carbohydrate metabolism and produce important thyroid hormones. Without enough manganese, our bodies cannot properly digest the foods we eat and we can't sustain optimal thyroid function, which, in turn, can lead to steady weight gain.

• **Plant sterols:** Most likely you've seen these healthy plant fats marketed on bottles of juice and tubs of margarine, which add sterols because science shows they can lower LDL ("bad") cholesterol by as much as 15 percent. But researchers say the outcome is far more effective when sterols are consumed by eating foods like nuts, which boast more naturally occurring sterols than most foods. While there is no specific research, per se, suggesting plant sterols help whittle down our waistlines, their cholesterol-lowering effect is so significant, it adds yet another reason to get your daily nut fix.

If you're the type of person to polish off a bowl of nuts at the bar, then you need to read this carefully: Adding nuts to your diet to lose weight *only* works if you adhere, give or take a few nuts, to about 1.5 ounces a day, the equivalent of a large handful. Since they are high in calories and fat, nuts will cause you to gain weight if you mindlessly overeat them, just as overeating almost any food does. If you have a problem with portion control, don't avoid nuts, but use them to garnish your morning oatmeal, afternoon yogurt, or dinner salad rather than eating them throughout the day as a snack. Or, if you do want to snack on nuts, preportion a few tablespoons into small baggies and never, ever eat straight from a jar or pouch.

2. NUTS ARE ONE OF THE MOST PLEASURABLE AND SATISFYING FAT-BURNING FOODS YOU CAN EAT.

It may sound contradictory, but you can rest assured it's absolutely true: Countless studies show eating more of one of the world's highest-fat, highest-calorie natural foods—nuts—can help people lose weight. Several large population studies have found that people who eat nuts weigh less and have smaller waists on average than those who don't eat nuts. Reams of research have also concluded that dieters who eat nuts lose more weight than nut avoiders. When study participants include small amounts of nuts in their daily diet, they are less likely to overeat and to stick with their diet plans longer than those who don't. In fact, according to a study published in the *American Journal of Clinical Nutrition*, dieters don't feel as though they're on a diet when they follow a plan, like the Greek Diet, that includes nuts. Another study, from Purdue University, found that when people ate an extra 250 calories per day in nuts, they didn't gain a single ounce more than those who ate fewer calories but no nuts.

Dry-Roasted, Oil-Roasted, or Raw?

Look for raw or dry-roasted nuts and seeds—those roasted in oil can contain more calories and unhealthy fats. Also, avoid sugar-coated nuts, whether homemade or store-bought: The amount of sugar used on these nuts undermines their waist-shrinking power.

How do nuts have this almost miraculous effect on weight loss? The answer is manifold. First, nuts are composed of mostly fat, and healthy fat is extremely satiating—unlike the unhealthy fat found in processed foods, which often increases hunger and triggers cravings. Nuts also taste rich, much richer than other high-fat, high-calorie foods like potato chips, which often just taste oily and salty (and are filled with unhealthy fats and chemicals). In addition, nuts provide an extremely sensory mouthfeel—crunchy on the outside, creamy on the inside—known to few other foods, especially snack foods. Lastly, nuts contain all the right macronutrients—fat, protein, and fiber—and are low in carbohydrates and high in micronutrients like vitamins and minerals shown to curb hunger and fire metabolism.

Finally, nuts have a special power found in few foods: Similar to prescription antidepressants, eating nuts increases levels of serotonin, the body's feel-good hormone. Not only does this make us happier and less irritable while we lose weight, serotonin has also been shown to reduce appetite and improve heart health.

The Lowdown on Nut Butters

Peanut butter and other nut and seed butters, like almond, cashew, and sunflower, are high in protein, but lack the fiber found in whole nuts and seeds. What's more, many commercial peanut butters contain added sugars. We recommend you opt only for 100 percent all-natural nut and seed butters, and use them in lieu of jam, jelly, and/or butter for a lower-sugar, more filling spread.

PILLAR TWELVE
Chicken and Eggs (Sensual)

WHEN I FIRST CAME TO NEW YORK IN 2011, I would go to the grocery store to buy the basics. The first time I was in the egg section, I was shocked by how many different varieties there were—medium, large, extra-large, organic, cage-free, free-range . . . the list goes on! I decided to buy half a dozen extra-large eggs, and half a dozen free-range eggs—I didn't know what the difference meant because, in Greece, an egg is an egg, especially at the village marketplace.

I quickly discovered something interesting. The regular extra-large eggs were *awful*! They had a terrible flavor and smell, and their yolks were light yellow. I had never seen an egg with a yolk that color. But then I cracked open one of the free-range eggs and saw something different—a rich, orange-colored yolk. This, I thought to myself, was an egg.

The experiment continued. When I started my restaurant in New York and had the difficult task of choosing the best vendors, I ordered a variety of different types of chicken from farms. I was sorely disappointed by all the conventional chicken, which had no flavor or taste. But the chicken labeled "organic" was completely different, full of character and so easy to cook with, just like the chicken I remember in Greece. And this character is so important. Yes, poultry is a blank canvas for whatever seasonings and sauces you add, but I believe every ingredient should have flavor that stands on its own—this way, you don't have to add as much seasonings and sauces!

POULTRY IN ANCIENT GREECE

There was really no such thing as what we know as a modern chicken in ancient Greece, as chickens were not domesticated until centuries later. The ancients did, however, have game birds like pheasant and quail, which they hunted and enjoyed as supplements to their plant-based diet. They also ate the eggs of these birds, but not as often as Westerners consume chicken and chicken eggs. As we've said, their diet was mostly plant-based, and they got plenty of protein from beans, whole grains, and, of course, fresh seafood.

GROWING UP WITH CHICKENS AND EGGS

My best friend growing up was named Kota-Kota. She was a chicken, and she would follow me *everywhere*. In the evening, when everyone would return from the farm after working all day in the fields, we would sit around the dinner table, and while Kota-Kota was supposed to be asleep with the rest of the chickens, she would instead be with me, resting by my feet or trying to climb into my lap, which was her favorite place. My mother and father didn't like me having a chicken for a pet because they worried I wouldn't eat eggs or chicken meat. But this wasn't the case! Although our family ate chicken only once a week, I ate eggs every day, in every way imaginable—for breakfast, lunch, and dinner.

In the winter, my grandmother and Aunt Maria would make *kotosoupa avgolemono,* or chicken soup with egg-lemon sauce, using the recipe passed down from my great-grandmother. (See my recipe on page 184.) My mother always reminded them to use the older chickens because their aged meat and bones made for a richer broth. They would boil the vegetables and chicken for six hours, skimming the fat off the top, to harness the flavor without all the fatty oils. Then, they added *hylopites,* or small square egg noodles, to bulk up the soup, along with the roots of dill and fennel for a wonderful flavor and aroma.

If my mother heard my siblings or me coughing when we came home from school, she would immediately give us a cup of chicken soup to ward off a cold. She always said it was the perfect food for any time, and none of us ever got very sick. I'm convinced it's because the chicken soup was so warming and hearty, and full of nutrients from three generations of homeopathic wisdom!

When it came to traditional avgolemono (egg-lemon sauce), my grandmother did not "rule the roost." She would make it from scratch every time we had soup because, for some reason, every time she made it ahead and tried to reheat it, it would curdle. As a young cook, I remember thinking there had to be an easier way to make it. Years later, I made it my mission to make the perfect avgolemono sauce, and I did!

Picking the Right Poultry Part

We believe all parts of a chicken—breasts, thighs, and drumsticks—should be included in a healthy weight-loss diet. Although dark-meat thighs and drumsticks are slightly higher in fat, they are also higher in certain nutrients like iron and can be more satisfying than leaner, white-meat chicken breasts. Also, chicken breasts don't work well in some dishes. As a good rule of thumb, you should choose chicken breasts for faster-cooking methods like pan-searing and grilling, opting for thighs and drumsticks for stewing, braising, and slow cooking.

CHICKEN AND EGGS TODAY

When I started cooking seriously, one of the first things I wanted to do was make my own avgolemono. I began experimenting to figure out the right proportions of ingredients and methods of cooking. After many attempts, I finally had the perfect recipe that tasted great, didn't curdle, and could be reheated over and over again. Best of all, it is so easy and versatile to use. Think of it as an easy, but healthier, hollandaise sauce—and you can pair it with everything. For my famous recipe, see page 276.

Today, I eat eggs nearly every morning, in countless different ways: hard-boiled, in omelets and frittatas, and "over medium." I love eggs because they're so filling. I eat two eggs in the morning and I don't feel hungry for hours. I love eating eggs for dinner, too, because they're easy to make and just as filling as other dinner foods. I wish more Americans thought of eggs as a dinner food because they make such beautiful, healthy, high-protein meals. Working fourteen to sixteen hours a day running around a kitchen takes a lot of energy. When I don't have enough protein, there's not enough Greek coffee in the world to wake me up. The simple addition of clean, organic protein, from either eggs or chickens, helps keep my energy up and my weight down.

I use eggs in many dishes, including in pastas, crab cakes, and lots of my desserts. Of course, my chicken dishes are also popular, and my signature lemon chicken (braised chicken in lemon–white wine sauce) is one of my best. In all these dishes, I only use organic, free-range chickens and eggs because, as I have learned, these ingredients are free of pesticides and antibiotics, which affect the flavor and taste of the dishes.

Chicken and Eggs (Science)

AS WE'VE SEEN, the traditional Greek diet is mostly plant-based, with plenty of fresh seafood on the side. But there's also a big place in our weekly diet for chicken and eggs, which is why we've included these power proteins as our twelfth Pillar Food. Both figure prominently in many classic Mediterranean dishes, including chicken soup and one of the tastiest (and healthiest) Greek sauces, *avgolemono,* which translates, literally, to "egg with lemon." Eating chicken and eggs prepared properly can help you lose weight and live healthier. Here's what you need to know about these foods:

1. THINK OF CHICKEN AS A SIDE DISH OR AN OCCASIONAL MAIN MEAL.

In ancient Greece, poultry was eaten on average once a week. The Greeks complemented their meals of vegetables, beans, and whole grains with a bit of pheasant or quail, but poultry was often seen as a side rather than the main meal.

The way the Greeks ate, along with anyone who follows a traditional Mediterranean diet today, is starkly different from most modern Western diets, in which chicken is often consumed daily, usually as the main dish for dinner, if not lunch, too. While many meals with chicken are healthy, depending on how we prepare them, prioritizing poultry as an everyday dish means we end up eating fewer plants and less fish and shellfish. The problem with this, as we've seen through the Pillars, is that both reams of research and history show eating more plants and seafood is the best way to lose weight and keep it off. By comparison, long-term and large-scale population studies suggest diets high in animal meat, including poultry, have been shown to increase the risk of obesity, along with cancer, heart disease, and other chronic modern illnesses.

That said, poultry still has a place in the Greek Diet and should be consumed the way the ancient Greeks did, eating chicken as a regular side or occasional main. Compared to red meat, chicken and turkey on average are lower in calories, cholesterol, and unhealthy saturated fat, but still pack lots of stomach-satiating protein, with 21 grams and 25 grams, respectively, for a 3-ounce serving of roasted chicken thigh and breast meat. In most recipes, cooking poultry with the skin on can increase the flavor of the meat, but be sure to remove the skin before consuming to keep calories and unhealthy fat in check.

WHEN IT COMES TO POULTRY PRODUCTS, ORGANIC MATTERS

If you can afford the price bump, organic poultry is a smart choice for you, the environment, and, surprisingly, your weight-loss efforts. Conventional chickens are given high levels of antibiotics and fed processed grain loaded with pesticides and fertilizers. These drugs and chemicals pass through to the meat, giving you a large dose of toxins that interfere with healthy hormone production and metabolism. What's more, studies show organic chicken is less likely to be contaminated with salmonella or contain arsenic, a harmful chemical found in soil and linked to an increased risk of cancer and heart disease.

Buying organic eggs is less important, because organic standards for eggs are generally not as robust as for poultry, allowing some organic producers to raise chickens in conditions below the standards for regular manufacturers. In addition, antibiotics and pesticides don't pass through to eggs. But choosing free-range or cage-free eggs ensures that chickens have more space to move and access to the outdoors, the more humane and healthier choices for both the chickens and the eggs. Free-range eggs, on average, have less cholesterol and saturated fat than conventional eggs, and are higher in healthy nutrients, including omega-3 fatty acids, vitamin E, and vitamin A.

Chicken Thighs for Thinner Thighs

Most people think of chicken breast as being the best cut for weight loss, but you should definitely not overlook thigh meat. While chicken thigh has slightly more calories and fat—a skinless thigh has 170 calories and 9 grams of fat, while a skinless breast has only 140 calories and 3 grams of fat—thigh meat's higher fat content can help fill you up for a very minimal difference in energy density. What's more, chicken thigh meat is richer and often tastier than breast meat, helping satisfy hunger. Finally, thigh meat contains higher concentrations of iron and zinc, minerals necessary for proper metabolism and immune function that women are often deficient in.

2. USE EGGS AS A PROTEIN SOURCE FOR BREAKFAST, LUNCH, AND DINNER TO HELP LOSE WEIGHT QUICKLY.

Eggs figure prominently in a traditional Greek Mediterranean diet, more so than chicken, because they're higher in vitamins, minerals, and antioxidants than animal meat. In just 85 calories, eggs pack lots of iron, zinc, and vitamins A, D, E, and B12, the latter an important nutrient for metabolism and energy and which overweight people are often low in. What's more, the protein found in eggs is the best-quality protein you can eat—superior to chicken breast or even red meat—with a higher concentration of essential amino acids that our bodies need for optimal function.

Because of their combination of high-quality protein and micronutrients, eggs make us feel fuller than other foods and can reduce cravings, according to research. A study from Louisiana State University found that women who ate two eggs every day for breakfast lost an incredible 65 percent more weight after 2 months than women who ate for breakfast a bagel of the same exact number of calories. Another study found that eating eggs instead of other foods reduces cravings for sugary and fatty food—a good reason to have an omelet for dinner if you tend to overeat at night.

Research also shows that eggs build muscle and increase strength more than other protein sources. Having more muscle not only helps you look better in a bathing suit, it also triggers quicker weight loss. Muscle burns more calories than fat, so the more muscle you're able to build in part by eating eggs, the more energy your body can burn at rest.

Finally, the high-quality protein and vitamins and minerals in eggs provide a sustained source of energy, helping you feel better throughout the day and giving you the jump you need to move more and exercise.

The Egg–Cholesterol Myth

Eggs have long been maligned for being high in cholesterol—each contains about 180 milligrams, or more than half the recommended daily amount (300 mg)—but a major analysis of past studies shows that eating an egg every day won't boost your risk of heart disease or stroke, as researchers previously thought. In fact, researchers found that having an egg daily may reduce the risk of heart disease, because eggs are high in nutrients that help promote heart health, including protein, vitamins B12 and D, riboflavin, and folate.

SUPPLEMENTAL FOODS

FOODS AND INGREDIENTS from the twelve Pillar Foods should make up the bulk of your diet. But sometimes a recipe or certain dish calls for the addition of what we call a supplemental food—those whole foods that aren't necessarily unhealthy, but that you don't want to eat on a regular basis. The following foods should be part of your diet no more than once a week, with the exception of Greek cheeses, which can be added to dishes in small amounts in moderation.

Honey: Whether you use table sugar, agave, molasses, or honey, all sweeteners have approximately the same number of calories and will spike your blood-sugar levels, especially if you consume them on their own or with other carbohydrates. But in comparison to all other sweeteners, honey is less refined and contains nutritional and medicinal benefits—just one reason nearly every ancient culture, including the Egyptians, Chinese, Mayans, Incas, and, of course, Greeks ate this food. In Greece, honey was ambrosia, a food of the twelve gods of Olympus, that also served as a potent medicine, capable of curing everything from deep cuts to sore throats to indigestion. Many believed that the more honey you consumed, the longer you lived. A sweet elixir, the ancient Greeks also cooked with honey, using the sweetener in breads, candy, and baklava, a dessert made out of nuts and phyllo pastry.

Today, science shows honey has strong medicinal purposes, capable of killing harmful bacteria, treating allergies, boosting immunity, and helping heal burns and other skin afflictions. More important for weight loss, research has also found honey helps control blood sugar levels and insulin sensitivity—a singular quality among sweeteners—making it the best choice for cooking and desserts. For recipes using honey, see page 265 for Honey Pie (Melopita), page 257 for Round Baklava, and page 180 for Salad with Orange-Honey Dressing.

Feta and Ricotta Cheeses: If there were to be a national cheese of Greece, it would be feta. This strongly flavored hard cheese stars in many dishes, but that's not a bad thing: Out of all cheeses, feta is lower in calories and has less fat than most, with a third fewer calories and less fat than cheddar. Feta also contains a good amount of protein and calcium, boasting 140 milligrams of the bone-building mineral per ounce. Calcium found naturally in foods like feta and Greek yogurt has been shown to stimulate fat breakdown and combat dangerous visceral, or abdominal, fat. What's more, research shows we eat smaller bites of food with a pungent smell like feta. For recipes containing feta, see page 226 for Scrambled Eggs with Feta Cheese (Kayana), page 177 for Greek Salad (Horiatiki Salata), and page 250 for Spring Stuffed Leg of Lamb (Boutaki Yemisto).

Ricotta was developed in Italy, but has been a part of traditional Mediterranean and Greek cooking for years. A soft cheese made from whey, ricotta is lower in fat than many hard cheeses like cheddar. Similar to feta, ricotta contains both calcium and protein, with approximately 15 grams in a half cup. All our recipes use *anthotyro,* a Greek form of ricotta that is naturally part skim. For recipes containing ricotta, see page 224 for Barley Rusks with Tomatoes (Dakos Me Domates), page 223 for Keftedes with Pligouri, and page 225 for Greek Frittata.

Phyllo: This thin pastry is a traditional delicacy in Greece, made from an unleavened dough of flour, water, and a small amount of olive oil and vinegar. Phyllo is lower in fat and calories than pie crust, tart shells, puff pastry, and many pizza crusts, making it an excellent and healthier alternative to all four. Unlike other pastry or bread doughs, phyllo comes in thin layers, so you can use as little as you please, creating a thin crust or shell for sweet or savory pies, pizza, and appetizers. The Fillo Factory sells several great varieties of organic, whole-grain phyllo dough. For recipes using phyllo, see page 206 for Spanakopita Triangles, page 208 for Wild Greens Pie (Hortopita), page 257 for Baklava, and page 207 for Pumpkin and Zucchini Pie (Kolokithopita).

Red Meat: The ancient Greeks didn't eat much red meat, but when they did, it was fresh lean meat from animals caught in the wild, like boar and deer, or that they raised on large expanses of farmland, such as goat and sheep. All the meat they ate was clean, meaning the animals were allowed to exercise, had exposure to fresh outdoor air, ate natural grasses, and were, of course, never exposed to artificial feed, hormones, steroids, or antibiotics.

By comparison, much of the cattle and sheep raised today are manufactured by large industrial meat producers, crowded into cramped indoor pens and paddocks, with little to no exposure to fresh air or exercise. They're fattened with a pesticide-rich grain feed, which their stomachs haven't evolved to eat, causing them to gain weight. Both cattle and sheep are given high doses of antibiotics to prevent the spread of disease in such cramped conditions, along with hormones and steroids so they grow larger and more quickly. The result is calorically dense, fatty cuts of meat high in pesticides, hormones, antibiotics, steroids, and other chemicals that can cause cancer and interfere with healthy hormone levels.

For this reason, if you want to eat beef or lamb once a week, it's imperative to choose a free-range grass-fed cut of meat, meaning the animal was allowed to pasture outdoors on grass. Ideally, the meat will not contain hormones, antibiotics, or steroids, but this cut can be difficult to find and costly when you do. Another choice is to eat game meat, such as bison, boar, and deer, all of which usually come from small ranchers who raise the animals in natural outdoor environments, with exposure to fresh air, exercise, and natural grass feed.

PART IV

THE RECIPES

SALADS

ROKA SALAD

I can't seem to get enough of this salad—the peppery flavor of arugula pairs beautifully with the slightly sweet, delightfully tart fig-balsamic vinaigrette; and the almonds add the crunch to balance it out just right.

SERVES 4

One 10-ounce bag prewashed arugula

3 dried figs, finely chopped

2 tablespoons (1 ounce) shaved Kefalograviera cheese or Pecorino Romano cheese

1 to 2 tablespoons (or 1 ounce) chopped almonds

Fig-Balsamic Dressing (recipe follows) or another dressing of your choice

1. In a large serving bowl, combine the arugula, figs, cheese, and almonds. Toss with a small amount of dressing until coated. Serve immediately.

Cook's note: If you opt for a different salad dressing, make sure it has either a Greek yogurt or olive oil base.

FIG-BALSAMIC DRESSING

MAKES ABOUT 1 CUP

¼ cup fig-infused balsamic vinegar or regular balsamic vinegar

1 teaspoon stoneground or Dijon mustard

2 dried figs, minced

¼ cup extra-virgin olive oil

Salt and freshly ground black pepper

1. In a food processor or blender, combine the balsamic vinegar, mustard, figs, and ¼ cup water. Blend for about 30 seconds or until the ingredients are well incorporated.

2. With the food processor or blender running, slowly add the olive oil in a thin stream. Blend until the dressing is emulsified. Season to taste with salt and pepper.

3. Transfer to an airtight container, cover tightly, and refrigerate for up to 2 weeks.

Cook's note: If you prefer a sweeter dressing, add a little more minced fig. If you like a spicier dressing, stir in a little additional mustard and freshly ground black pepper.

MAROULI SALAD

This verdant winter salad is a favorite of mine—I eat it all the time! Make it and serve with the feta-yogurt dressing, or dress it with a touch of olive oil and vinegar, and enjoy!

SERVES 4

3 hearts of romaine, cut into thin shreds or strips (chiffonade)
½ bunch fresh dill, stemmed and finely chopped
1 bunch scallions (white and light-green parts only), thinly sliced
Feta-Yogurt Dressing (recipe follows)
Crumbled feta cheese, for topping

1. In a large bowl, toss together the romaine, dill, and scallions. Toss with a small amount of dressing until coated. Top with crumbled feta.

FETA-YOGURT DRESSING

MAKES 1 CUP

2 tablespoons crumbled feta cheese

2 tablespoons 2% plain Greek yogurt

2 tablespoons finely chopped fresh dill

1 tablespoon red wine vinegar

¼ teaspoon mustard powder

2 tablespoons olive oil

Salt and freshly ground black pepper

Dried oregano

1. In a medium bowl, combine the feta, yogurt, dill, vinegar, and mustard powder. Pour in the olive oil and whisk until it is thoroughly incorporated. Taste the dressing and season to taste with salt, pepper, and oregano.

COUSCOUS SALAD

This salad embodies the spirit of the Mediterranean, but is light and bright. The use of whole-grain couscous increases the fiber content, and gives a rougher, more appealing texture.

SERVES 3 TO 4

1 cup vegetable stock or water

1 cup whole-grain couscous

1 tablespoon Greek olive oil

Salt

½ cup 2% plain Greek yogurt

10 cherry tomatoes, halved

1 bunch fresh flat-leaf parsley, stemmed and finely chopped

3 tablespoons finely chopped fresh mint leaves (no stems)

½ cup finely chopped red, green, yellow, or orange bell peppers

4 teaspoons white wine vinegar

Juice of 1 lemon

1. In a medium saucepan, bring the vegetable stock to a boil. Stir in the couscous, olive oil, and salt to taste. Cover the saucepan with a kitchen towel (this helps the couscous to cook and get fluffy), put on the lid, and set aside off the heat until all the liquid is absorbed, 10 to 15 minutes. Fluff the couscous with a fork.

2. Transfer the couscous to a large bowl. Stir in the yogurt, cherry tomatoes, parsley, mint, bell pepper, vinegar, and lemon juice. Cover and refrigerate for at least 20 minutes so the flavors can blend.

LENTIL SALAD WITH ORANGES

Protein-packed and colorful, this lentil salad is great on its own or paired with Grilled Chicken Breast (page 246). Feel free to add your favorite vegetables or a different citrus fruit to make it your own!

SERVES 4 TO 6

2 cups lentils (preferably brown or red)
Salt and freshly ground black pepper
4 or 5 scallions (white and light-green parts only), sliced
1 medium red onion, sliced
1 cucumber, diced
1 red bell pepper, sliced
1 red apple, unpeeled, diced
2 oranges, peeled and sliced
½ bunch fresh flat-leaf parsley, stemmed and chopped
½ cup olive oil
Juice of 1 orange
White wine vinegar

1. Rinse the lentils. In a saucepan, cover the lentils with lightly salted water, bring to a boil over medium heat, and cook until tender, about 50 minutes. Drain the lentils and allow them to cool.

2. In a large bowl, combine the scallions, red onion, cucumber, bell pepper, apple, oranges, parsley, olive oil, orange juice, and salt, pepper, and vinegar to taste.

3. Stir in the lentils and mix well. Set the salad aside for about 10 minutes before serving so that the flavors can develop.

GREEK SALAD (HORIATIKI SALATA)

Horiatiki salata is the iconic Greek salad everyone knows and loves. Perfect for lunch, dinner, or a snack in between, this salad fills you up without weighing you down.

SERVES 3 TO 4

2 medium tomatoes, cut into wedges

1 medium red onion, sliced or cut into pieces

1 green bell pepper, cut into rounds or sliced

¾ cucumber, sliced (reserve the remaining cucumber for the dressing)

¼ cup pitted kalamata olives

¼ cup crumbled feta cheese

Salt and freshly ground black pepper

Dakos (optional; see Cook's note)

Cucumber Dressing (recipe follows) or another dressing, preferably with a Greek yogurt or olive oil base

Fresh oregano leaves, for garnish

1. In a large bowl, combine the tomatoes, red onion, bell pepper, cucumber, olives, and feta. Sprinkle to taste with salt and pepper. Add the *dakos* (if using). Toss with a small amount of the dressing until coated. Sprinkle with oregano and serve immediately.

Cook's note: Dakos are Greek barley rusks that are usually sold dried and are often used in Greek cooking as a textural component; they are a great source of fiber. While you may substitute well-toasted pieces of dense, whole-grain or multigrain bread in a pinch, the barley rusks are better. If you cannot locate them in a local shop, barley rusks may be ordered online.

CUCUMBER DRESSING

MAKES ABOUT 1 CUP

¼ cucumber, peeled

1½ teaspoons fresh lemon juice

2 tablespoons minced fresh flat-leaf parsley leaves (no stems)

2 tablespoons capers, rinsed

½ teaspoon dried oregano

½ cup olive oil

Salt and freshly ground black pepper

1. In a blender or food processor, combine the cucumber, lemon juice, parsley, capers, and oregano. Blend for 30 to 60 seconds, or until smooth. With the blender running, slowly add the olive oil and blend until emulsified. Add salt and pepper to taste.

2. Transfer the dressing to an airtight container, cover, and refrigerate for up to 1 week. Shake the dressing before using it to combine all the ingredients.

POMEGRANATE-KALE SALAD

This superfood salad is packed full of antioxidants, which makes it healthy, but what I love about it is the texture of the raw kale and crunch of the pomegranate seeds.

SERVES 4 TO 6

1 pound kale, torn into bite-size pieces

Seeds from 1 pomegranate (½ to 1 cup)

Salt and freshly ground black pepper

1 cup olive oil

¼ cup white wine vinegar

¼ cup honey

1. In a large bowl, combine the kale and pomegranate seeds. Season with salt and pepper to taste.

2. In a small bowl, whisk together the oil, vinegar, and honey until well combined. Pour the dressing onto the kale and pomegranate seeds until they are evenly coated.

TUNA SALAD (TONOSALATA)

Tuna salad, as Americans know it, is full of mayonnaise, lacking character and flavor. My version is closer to the French-Mediterranean Niçoise version—light and fresh, highlighting the tuna, accented with fresh lemon. Eat this for a satisfying lunch, or pair it with some whole-grain pasta for a nutritious dinner.

SERVES 2

1 large romaine heart, sliced
2 scallions, sliced (white and light-green parts only)
3 tablespoons chopped fresh dill leaves (no stems)
10 cherry tomatoes, halved
½ cup cooked corn kernels
2 teaspoons white wine vinegar
One 7-ounce can tuna (packed in water or olive oil)
Salt and freshly ground black pepper
2 tablespoons olive oil
Juice of 1 lemon

1. In a large bowl, toss together the romaine, scallions, dill, cherry tomatoes, corn, and vinegar. Mix well and plate.

2. Season the tuna with salt and pepper. Place the tuna on top of the vegetables and drizzle with the olive oil and lemon juice.

SALAD WITH ORANGE-HONEY DRESSING

This citrus-centric salad is a wonderful way to brighten up any meal! Pair it with a bowl of Lentil Soup (page 186) or some Grilled Calamari (page 241) for a great meal!

SERVES 4 TO 6

3 romaine hearts, chopped
3 small zucchini, grated
2 carrots, grated
1 small tomato, diced
½ bunch fresh flat-leaf parsley, stemmed and finely chopped
1 navel (or another variety) orange, separated into segments

FOR THE DRESSING
2 tablespoons olive oil
1 tablespoon honey
Grated zest of 1 orange
½ cup fresh orange juice (about 2 oranges)
Salt and freshly ground black pepper

1. In a large salad bowl, toss together the romaine, zucchini, carrots, tomato, parsley, and orange segments.

2. For the dressing: In a small bowl, whisk together the olive oil, honey, orange zest, and orange juice.

3. Pour the dressing over the salad and toss so that all the vegetables are evenly coated with dressing. Season to taste with salt and pepper.

WHEAT BERRY SALAD

I remember during the wheat harvest my aunt would make this salad, and for months it was all that I talked about. I love the crunchy texture of the nuts and pomegranate seeds. Eat this for lunch with some homemade or store-bought Greek yogurt.

SERVES 4 TO 6

½ pound wheat berries (1¼ cups)
½ cup whole roasted blanched almonds
½ cup chopped walnuts
1 tablespoon sesame seeds
Seeds from 1 pomegranate
1 tablespoon chopped fresh flat-leaf parsley leaves (no stems)
½ teaspoon ground cinnamon
¼ teaspoon ground cloves
½ cup raisins
Salt

1. The night before you plan to serve this salad, place the wheat berries in a large bowl with water to cover by 1 inch. Cover the bowl and set aside to soak overnight.

2. The next day, drain the wheat berries into a large colander. Transfer them to a medium saucepan and add enough water to cover by 2 inches. Cover and cook over medium-low heat until plump and tender, about 2 hours.

3. Drain the wheat berries. Spread them out on a baking sheet lined with a kitchen towel. Set aside for 25 to 30 minutes, tossing occasionally, to allow them to drain and dry out.

4. In a large bowl, combine the wheat berries, almonds, walnuts, sesame seeds, pomegranate seeds, parsley, cinnamon, cloves, raisins, and salt to taste. Mix well to combine. Refrigerate the salad, covered, for about 2 hours so the flavors and aromas will blend. Taste and add salt as needed before serving.

FRUIT SALAD

Eating a piece of fresh fruit is a great way to enjoy the nutritional benefits from one fruit, but eating fruit salad allows you to enjoy the benefits from all the fruits you use. Feel free to add your favorite fruits to this delicious, healthy treat!

SERVES 4 TO 6

2 pears (any variety), peeled and cut into bite-size pieces
Seeds from 1 pomegranate
8 strawberries, hulled and sliced
8 to 12 cherries, pitted
1 bunch seedless green or red grapes (1 to 2 cups)
1 cup walnuts or whole blanched almonds
¼ to ½ teaspoon ground cinnamon
1 cup fresh orange juice (about 3 oranges)
1 tablespoon honey
Greek yogurt, for garnish

1. In a large bowl, combine the pears, pomegranate seeds, strawberries, cherries, and grapes. Add the walnuts and cinnamon, and toss to combine.

2. In a small bowl, whisk together the orange juice and honey. Pour the mixture over the fruit salad and toss to coat the fruit evenly. Cover and refrigerate for 15 to 20 minutes to allow the flavors to marry. Serve the fruit salad with a dollop of Greek yogurt.

WATERMELON SALAD WITH FETA AND MINT

Perhaps the most refreshing of all dishes, this watermelon and feta salad is perfect for a hot summer day. Enjoy this on its own for a light lunch, or as a slightly savory dessert after some souvlaki (see recipes on pages 192, 239, 245, and 254).

SERVES 4

2 cups cubed watermelon (1- to 2-inch cubes)
⅓ cup diced or crumbled feta cheese
½ cup raisins
20 fresh mint leaves
Honey and/or crushed nuts of your choice (optional)

1. In a large bowl, combine the watermelon and feta. Add the raisins and mint and stir to combine. Cover the bowl with plastic wrap and refrigerate for 15 to 20 minutes to allow the flavors to marry.

2. Serve the salad as is, or with a drizzle of honey and/or a sprinkle of nuts.

SOUPS

CHICKEN SOUP WITH EGG-LEMON EMULSION (KOTOSOUPA AVGOLEMONO)

The ultimate panacea, this chicken soup feeds your heart and soul, in addition to your stomach. Perfect for curing any ailment, this recipe is exactly how my grandmother used to make it for me, but if you like, feel free to add other vegetables and herbs that you enjoy!

SERVES 8 TO 10

1 whole chicken (3 to 4 pounds), skin removed
1 medium red onion, chopped
2 celery stalks, chopped
¼ cup olive oil
Salt and freshly ground black pepper
½ cup Loi Kritharaki Orzo Pasta (or another whole-grain pasta)
Egg-Lemon (Avgolemono) Sauce (page 276)
Chopped fresh parsley, for garnish
Lemon wedges, for garnish

1. Rinse the chicken well and place it in a large pot. Add water to cover the chicken by 1 or 2 inches. Add the onion, celery, olive oil, and salt and pepper to taste. Bring to a boil, reduce to a simmer until the chicken is tender and thoroughly cooked, 35 to 40 minutes. If the liquid no longer completely covers the chicken as it cooks, add a little more.

2. Remove the chicken from the pot and place it on a large platter. When cool enough to handle, pull the meat from the bones and cut into tiny pieces or shred it by hand. Cover the platter of meat with foil and set aside.

3. Strain the broth from cooking the chicken through a large sieve set over a large bowl (reserve the onion and celery). Measure the number of cups of broth. You will need 8 cups of liquid, so add water if you need to.

4. Pour the broth back into the pot. Return the onion and the celery to the broth. Bring the broth to a boil over medium heat. When the broth boils, stir in the pasta. Continue to boil over medium heat, stirring, until the pasta is al dente or cooked to desired doneness.

5. Remove the pot from the heat and stir in the reserved chicken pieces. Stir in the avgolemono sauce and continue stirring until it is fully incorporated. Return the soup to low heat and cook, stirring, for about 1 minute.

6. Serve the soup garnished with fresh parsley and lemon wedges.

PEA AND LEEK SOUP (HORTOSOUPA)

One of my springtime favorites, this pea and leek soup is bursting with vegetables and full of flavor. If you like, finish it with a touch of tangy Greek yogurt. Served hot or cold, it never fails to put a smile on my face and a "spring" in my step!

SERVES 8 TO 10

2 cups chopped leeks, white and light-green parts only (about 2 leeks)
1 cup chopped yellow onion
Salt and freshly ground black pepper
4 cups vegetable stock
5 cups shelled fresh peas or two 10-ounce packages frozen peas
⅔ cup chopped fresh mint leaves (no stems)
½ cup 2% plain Greek yogurt (see Cook's note)
½ cup chopped fresh chives

1. Heat a large saucepan over medium heat for about 5 minutes, or until very hot. Add the leeks and onion to the pan and cook over medium heat until the onions are translucent and softened, 5 to 10 minutes. About halfway through the cooking, sprinkle the vegetables with salt to draw out the moisture. (Drawing out the moisture helps reduce the cooking time.)

2. Pour in the vegetable stock, increase the heat to medium-high, and bring the soup to a boil. Stir in the peas and cook until the peas are tender, 3 to 5 minutes. Remove the saucepan from the heat, stir in the mint, and sprinkle with salt and pepper to taste.

3. Using a blender set on low speed, puree the soup in batches, blending about 1 cup at a time, and transferring to a large bowl as you work. Whisk in the yogurt, chives, and additional salt and pepper, if desired.

4. To serve the soup hot, reheat it over high heat, stirring to prevent sticking. To serve the soup cold, refrigerate, tightly covered, until it is well chilled.

Cook's note: As an alternative to adding the Greek yogurt to the soup, you may serve it on the side as a garnish or omit it entirely for a vegan soup.

LENTIL SOUP (FAKES)

Many cultures have their version of lentil soup—what I love the most about mine is the simplicity of the soup, and the way the flavor and texture of the lentil doesn't get marred or lost in a sea of ingredients. Eat this with a Marouli Salad (page 174) for a heart-healthy lunch or dinner.

SERVES 6 TO 8

Salt and freshly ground black pepper
1 pound lentils (any kind, though brown/black are best for this soup)
1 medium red onion, finely chopped
1 garlic clove, minced
2 carrots, sliced into rounds
2 tomatoes, grated (on the large holes of a box grater)
1 teaspoon tomato paste
1 bay leaf
1 sprig of fresh rosemary
⅓ cup olive oil

1. In a large pot, bring 8 cups lightly salted water to a boil. Stir in the lentils and simmer them until slightly hydrated, 10 to 15 minutes. Drain the lentils into a large colander and discard the cooking liquid.

2. In a large saucepan over medium heat, sauté the onion until golden and softened, 5 minutes. Stir in the lentils, garlic, carrots, grated tomato, tomato paste, bay leaf, rosemary, and salt and pepper to taste. Stir in 8 cups water, bring to a boil, and simmer until the lentils are soft, 35 to 45 minutes.

3. Slowly add the olive oil, stirring continuously, and simmer the soup for 10 to 15 more minutes, or until it thickens. Taste and add salt and pepper as desired. Remove the bay leaf and the rosemary sprig before serving.

MUSHROOM BARLEY SOUP

Earthy and hearty, this soup will warm you and fill you up on a cold day. Feel free to add your favorite mushrooms to the mix, or some garlic to spice it up a bit.

SERVES 12

1 cup hulled or pearled barley
1 medium red onion, finely chopped
Salt and freshly ground black pepper
¼ cup olive oil
½ pound mushrooms (button, cremini, portobello), sliced
½ cup white wine
6 cups vegetable stock or water
½ bunch fresh flat-leaf parsley, stemmed and finely chopped

1. The night before you plan to serve the soup, place the barley in a large bowl with water to cover by 2 to 3 inches. Set aside to soak overnight.

2. The following day, drain the barley, transfer it to a large pot, and add enough water to cover by 2 to 3 inches. Bring to a boil, reduce to a simmer and cook until the barley is al dente, about 40 minutes. You'll be cooking it longer in the soup itself, so you don't want it to be mushy. Drain the barley.

3. In a large, dry saucepan, sauté the onion with a pinch of salt over medium heat until golden brown and softened, 8 to 10 minutes. Add the olive oil and when it is very hot, stir in the mushrooms and sauté them until they are nicely browned, 3 to 4 minutes.

4. Add the drained barley to the saucepan and stir until it is well combined with the onion and mushrooms. Deglaze the saucepan with the wine, allowing the alcohol to evaporate. Pour the stock into the saucepan and simmer the soup on low heat for about 35 minutes. Add the parsley, and salt and pepper to taste. Continue to cook for 10 minutes, or until the soup is cooked to your liking and all the ingredients are blended together nicely.

5. Serve the soup as is, or, for a creamier version, puree 2 cups of the soup in a blender or food processer, transfer it back to the saucepan, and stir to combine. Return the soup to a boil, then remove from the heat and serve.

GREEK FISH STEW (KAKAVIA)

This fisherman's stew comes from a long tradition of using the catch of the day to feed a ship's crew with only the ingredients available. Though nowadays there are many different types of fish on hand, keeping the ingredients to a minimum upholds the principles this dish is based on.

SERVES 2 TO 4

2 tablespoons olive oil
1 large onion, diced
2 garlic cloves, thinly sliced
3 celery stalks, sliced crosswise
2 bay leaves
2 medium tomatoes, diced
2 carrots, sliced crosswise into rounds
1 cup white wine
Salt and freshly ground black pepper
Two 8- to 10-ounce cod or monkfish fillets
4 to 5 tablespoons fresh lemon juice (about 2 lemons)
1 tablespoon chopped fresh dill leaves (no stems)
1 tablespoon chopped fresh flat-leaf parsley leaves (no stems)
Crusty multigrain bread, for serving (optional)

1. Heat a medium soup pot over medium heat until very hot. Add the olive oil and heat until it's very hot. Add the onion, garlic, and celery, and sauté until the vegetables are softened, 3 or 4 minutes.

2. Stir in the bay leaves, tomatoes, and carrots, and sauté for another 3 to 4 minutes. Pour in the wine and enough water so the liquid just covers the vegetables (about 4 cups). Cook over medium heat until the carrots are soft, 10 to 15 minutes. Season with pepper to taste.

3. Arrange the fish fillets over the vegetables, cover the pot, and cook until the fish is cooked through, another 10 minutes. Add 3 tablespoons lemon juice, taste the broth, and adjust the seasoning with more lemon juice, and some salt if needed.

4. Serve sprinkled with the dill and parsley, with crusty multigrain bread on the side if desired.

Cook's note: The salt used in this recipe is very minimal for a few reasons. The addition of celery reduces the need for extra salt. The lemon adds a beautiful bright acid that cuts the need for extra salt, and the fish itself is naturally salty and infuses the broth with fish flavor and salinity.

TAHINI VEGETABLE SOUP (TAHINOSOUPA)

This soup warms you up from the inside out! Excellent for a cold winter's night, with the added benefit and flavor of all the nutrients that sesame seeds (and their paste, tahini) have to offer. If you're feeling adventurous, add some of your favorite fresh herbs before you serve, and enjoy! This soup can also be refrigerated and served chilled with a dollop of yogurt—great for the summer!

SERVES 6 TO 8

1 medium potato, peeled and cut into medium chunks
2 carrots, cut into medium rounds
2 medium red onions, chopped
Salt and freshly ground black pepper
2 bunches Swiss chard, trimmed and chopped
2 celery stalks, chopped
1 cup orzo
5 tablespoons tahini (sesame paste)
Juice of 1 lemon
Finely chopped fresh flat-leaf parsley, for garnish

1. In a large pot, combine the potato, carrots, onions, and 8 cups water. Sprinkle with a little salt, bring to a boil over medium heat, and cook until the vegetables are tender, 30 to 40 minutes.

2. Stir in the Swiss chard and celery and cook for another 5 minutes.

3. Reserving the broth, strain the vegetables into a colander set over a large bowl. Transfer the vegetables to a food processor or blender and puree.

4. Pour the broth back into the pot and bring to a boil over medium-high heat. Stir in the orzo and season to taste with salt and pepper. Cook the orzo until al dente, 10 to 12 minutes. Return the pureed vegetables to the pot and stir well to combine. Cook the soup for another 2 minutes. Remove the soup from the heat and set aside for a few minutes so that the flavors will marry.

5. In a medium bowl, combine the tahini, lemon juice, and ⅓ cup of the soup. Stir very well to combine. Gradually stir the tahini mixture back into the pot. Serve the soup garnished with parsley.

Cook's note: In order to prevent curdling and to ensure a smoothly textured soup, it's important to temper the tahini–lemon juice mixture. Do this by gradually adding a little of the hot soup to the tahini–lemon juice mixture and then whisking thoroughly before adding it to the pot.

CHICKPEA STEW (SIFNOS REVITHADA)

This rustic chickpea stew hails from the island of Sifnos, where they cook it in a clay pot the night before the Sunday family supper. Eat this with a Greek Salad (Horiatiki Salata, see page 177) and some Whole-Grain Pita Bread (page 280), and you'll feel like you're in Sifnos!

SERVES 4 TO 6

1 pound dried chickpeas
1 teaspoon baking soda
2 medium red onions, finely chopped
½ cup olive oil
½ bunch fresh flat-leaf parsley, stemmed and finely chopped
½ bunch fresh dill, stemmed and finely chopped
Salt and freshly ground black pepper
Fresh lemon juice, for serving

1. The night before you plan to serve the stew, put the chickpeas in a large pot with water to cover by 1 inch. Stir in the baking soda, cover, and soak overnight.

2. The next day, drain and rinse the chickpeas. Transfer them to a Dutch oven or other large pot. Add the onions, olive oil, parsley, dill, salt and pepper to taste, and water to cover.

3. Preheat the oven to 300°F.

4. Cover and bake for about 6 hours, removing the cover in the last 30 minutes to allow the excess liquid to evaporate. Remove the chickpea stew from the oven, let it stand for a few minutes, and stir in fresh lemon juice to taste.

Cook's note: If you want this dish to be ready faster, you may bake it at 375°F for about 1½ hours instead. However, this yields a slightly less robust flavor profile.

CANNELLINI BEAN SOUP (FASOLADA)

Sometimes referred to as the "national food of the Greeks," *fasolada* holds a special place in every Greek child's heart. Made with the most basic ingredients, this soup reminds us all of home.

SERVES 4

1 pound dried cannellini beans
8 cups lukewarm water
3 medium tomatoes, grated (on the large holes of a box grater)
2 medium red onions, finely chopped
2 carrots, cut crosswise into ½-inch rounds
1 teaspoon tomato paste
¼ cup olive oil
1 red chile pepper, finely chopped
2 celery stalks, chopped
2 tablespoons finely chopped fresh flat-leaf parsley leaves (no stems), and more for garnish
Salt and freshly ground black pepper

1. The night before you plan to serve the soup, place the beans in a large pot with enough water to cover by 2 or 3 inches. (Soaking overnight will shorten the cooking time the next day.)

2. On the following day, drain the beans. Add them to a large pot and cover with water. Cook the beans, uncovered, for 30 minutes, skimming the surface occasionally to remove any foam. Drain the beans and discard the cooking water.

3. Return the beans to the pot, add the lukewarm water, and bring to a boil. Stir in the tomatoes, onions, and carrots. Stir the tomato paste into the olive oil. Stir this mixture into the pot of beans and vegetables. Cook the soup over medium heat, stirring occasionally, for 30 minutes.

4. Stir in the chile, celery, parsley, and salt and pepper to taste. Continue to boil over medium heat until the beans and vegetables are tender, another 20 minutes.

5. Serve the soup garnished with parsley.

VEGETARIAN

VEGETABLE SOUVLAKI

Souvlaki is a classic Greek dish of small pieces of food grilled on a wooden skewer. What's great about this vegetable souvlaki is that it's hearty and filling without the calories and saturated fat of animal meat.

SERVES 6 TO 8

½ cup Greek olive oil, plus more for drizzling

1 garlic clove, crushed

½ bunch finely chopped fresh flat-leaf parsley leaves (no stems)

One 250-gram package halloumi cheese, cut into 2-inch cubes

10 cherry tomatoes

1 medium red onion, cut into 2-inch pieces

1 medium eggplant, cut into 2-inch cubes

1 medium green bell pepper, cut into 2-inch pieces

1 medium zucchini, cut into 2-inch cubes

Dried oregano

Salt and freshly ground black pepper

Whole-grain pita bread, optional

1. Soak some 10-inch wooden skewers in water to cover for about 1 hour (this will prevent them from burning on the grill). If you use metal skewers, skip to step 2.

2. In a large bowl, combine the olive oil, garlic, and parsley. Add the halloumi, cherry tomatoes, onion, eggplant, bell pepper, and zucchini. Toss to coat with the olive oil. Cover the bowl and refrigerate for 30 minutes.

3. Thread the vegetables and the halloumi on the skewers, starting with a piece of red onion, then a piece of bell pepper, a cherry tomato, a cube of halloumi, a cube of eggplant, and a cube of zucchini. Continue this process until all the skewers are full. Drizzle them with a little olive oil and season them with salt, black pepper, and oregano to taste.

4. Preheat a grill to high or preheat a grill pan over high heat until it is very hot. Grill the skewers for about 2 minutes per side, or until the vegetables are as done as you like. Allow the souvlaki to rest for a few minutes before serving.

5. Heat the pitas on the grill or warm them in a preheated 325°F oven for 5 to 7 minutes. Take the vegetables and halloumi off the skewers and serve in the pita.

VEGETABLE STEW (TURLU)

A hearty and healthy stew that's versatile enough to let you switch up the vegetables according to their seasons. It's important to remember that not all vegetables take the same amount of time to cook, so the order of adding ingredients can vary depending on what you use.

SERVES 8 TO 10

1½ pounds zucchini (2 medium), cut into 4 x ½-inch strips

1 pound eggplant (1 large), cut into 4 x ½-inch strips

Salt and freshly ground black pepper

3 carrots, cut into 2-inch lengths

2 green bell peppers, cut into eighths

2 medium Yukon Gold potatoes (about ¾ pound total), peeled and chunked

1 red onion, cut into ½-inch-thick slices

¼ cup extra-virgin olive oil

2 garlic cloves, thinly sliced

¼ teaspoon ground allspice

2 tablespoons tomato paste

2 cups tomato puree

½ cup roughly chopped fresh flat-leaf parsley leaves (no stems)

½ cup roughly chopped fresh dill leaves (no stems)

1. Place the zucchini and the eggplant in separate bowls and sprinkle each bowlful with about 1 teaspoon of salt; toss well. Transfer both to a colander in the sink for about 30 minutes. Rinse the vegetables under cold running water to remove the salt and pat them dry with paper towels.

2. Preheat the oven to 425°F.

3. In a large roasting pan, toss the eggplant, carrots, bell peppers, potatoes, onion, olive oil, garlic, and allspice. Season with salt and pepper to taste. Roast the vegetables for about 35 minutes, stirring every 15 minutes, until they are golden and look roasted. Stir in the zucchini and roast for an additional 15 minutes.

4. In a small bowl, stir together the tomato paste and tomato puree. Stir this into the roasted vegetables. Continue roasting the vegetables for another 15 minutes to allow the flavors to marry.

5. Remove the stew from the oven, stir in the dill and parsley, and season with salt and pepper if necessary. Serve the stew warm.

Cook's note: This dish lends itself to variations. It's a seasonal dish, and you should use whatever vegetables are in season at the time. The recipe here is perfect for the beginning of autumn; in the winter, make it with butternut squash and Brussels sprouts or turnips in place of the zucchini and eggplant.

VEGETARIAN MOUSSAKA

A wonderful alternative to the classic Greek meat version, this moussaka is full of flavor and texture, while still being incredible nutritious and tasty! Eat this with a piece of Wild Greens Pie (page 208) for an amazing vegetarian dinner!

SERVES 12

FOR THE BOTTOM LAYER

2 or 3 Sicilian eggplants (or regular eggplant)

Olive oil, for brushing

Salt and freshly ground black pepper

FOR THE FILLING

5 white onions

2 pounds button mushrooms

2 medium zucchini

2 tomatoes

3 tablespoons tomato paste

¼ cup olive oil

1 cinnamon stick

2 bay leaves

½ cup red wine

Salt and freshly ground black pepper

½ cup Caramelized Tomatoes (and Coulis) (page 277)

FOR THE TOPPING

Mashed Cauliflower with Roasted Garlic (page 203)

About 2 tablespoons poppyseeds

1. Preheat the oven to 375°F. Line a baking sheet with parchment paper.

2. Prepare the bottom layer: Wash the eggplants and cut crosswise into ¼- to ½-inch-thick slices. Brush both sides of the slices with olive oil. Season lightly with salt and pepper. Bake the eggplant for 15 to 20 minutes, or until lightly golden and cooked through. Remove the eggplant from the oven and set aside.

3. Prepare the filling: Cut the onions into large pieces, and pulse them in a food processor so that they are chopped but not mushy. (Alternatively, dice the onions by hand.)

4. In a pot large enough to comfortably hold all the vegetables, sauté the onion over medium heat until softened, adding a pinch of salt to draw out the moisture.

5. Wash the mushrooms and pulse them in the food processor until they are chopped, being careful to avoid overprocessing and making them mushy. (Alternatively, you may chop the mushrooms by hand.) Chop the zucchini and the tomatoes together in the food processor (or by hand).

6. Add the zucchini, mushrooms, and tomatoes to the onion mixture and stir well. Cook over medium heat, stirring occasionally, until most of the liquid from the vegetables has evaporated. Stir in the tomato paste and olive oil, mixing thoroughly, and continue cooking until caramelized, another 5 to 10 minutes.

7. Reduce the heat to low, add the cinnamon stick and bay leaves, and deglaze with the wine. Continue to cook, stirring to make sure the filling doesn't stick to the bottom of the pan, until the wine has been absorbed by the vegetables. Remove the pot from the heat and set aside.

8. To assemble the moussaka, thin the tomato coulis with 2 or 3 tablespoons water. Spread the tomato coulis in the bottom of a 9 x 13-inch baking pan. Cover the coulis with baked eggplant slices, overlapping slightly to create a bed of eggplant for the filling. Repeat to make 2 layers of eggplant on the bottom.

9. Spread the filling over the eggplant layer evenly. It should be about 1½ inches thick. Be careful not to pack it too tightly or it won't be light and fluffy!

10. Top the moussaka with mashed cauliflower, spreading it out to create an even layer. Sprinkle with poppyseeds, and bake for 20 to 30 minutes, or until the top is golden brown. Remove the moussaka from the oven and let it rest for 10 to 15 minutes before serving.

ARTICHOKE STEW WITH VEGETABLES (ARTICHOKES "A LA POLITA")

Known as a "city-style" dish (*a la polita*) and harkening from the days of Constantinople, this artichoke-vegetable stew is now simple enough for people living in cities today to make easily. If you add Egg-Lemon (Avgolemono) Sauce (page 276) to this recipe, the finished dish is exactly how my grandmother used to make it.

SERVES 8

8 artichokes
Juice of 1 lemon plus ¼ cup more
2 medium red onions, finely chopped
4 scallions (white and light-green parts only), finely chopped
4 carrots, cut crosswise into ½-inch rounds
2 medium potatoes, peeled and diced
Salt and freshly ground black pepper
1 bunch fresh dill, stemmed and finely chopped
3 tablespoons olive oil

1. Remove the hard outer leaves of each artichoke by pulling them down toward the stem. Once you reach the softer inner leaves, cut off the hard top from the artichoke and remove the "choke" (the hairy innards) with a teaspoon. Cut the stem off, leaving ½ inch at the bottom, and halve the artichokes lengthwise. Place them in a bowl filled with water and the juice of 1 lemon (this will help keep the artichokes from discoloring). Drain well.

2. In a large saucepan over medium heat, sauté the onions until softened, 7 to 9 minutes. Stir in the scallions, carrots, potatoes, and artichokes, and continue to cook until everything looks caramelized, 7 to 8 minutes.

3. Stir in the ¼ cup lemon juice, 2 cups water, and salt and pepper to taste. Bring the mixture to a boil and cook over medium heat until all the vegetables are tender, about 30 minutes.

4. Stir in the dill and olive oil, and continue to cook for 10 more minutes. Remove from the heat and adjust the seasonings with salt and pepper as needed before serving.

STUFFED BABY EGGPLANT (PAPOUTSAKIA)

The decadent flavor and texture of perfectly cooked eggplant paired with the vegetable medley and the richness of my house-made Greek yogurt makes this one of my favorites.

SERVES 10

FOR THE FILLING

1 red bell pepper, finely diced

1 green bell pepper, finely diced

1 yellow bell pepper, finely diced

1 zucchini, finely diced

1 carrot, finely diced

1 white onion, finely diced

1 medium red onion, finely diced

Salt and freshly ground black pepper

1 heaping tablespoon tomato paste

4 to 5 tablespoons Caramelized Tomatoes (and Coulis) (page 277)

FOR THE EGGPLANT

10 baby eggplants

Olive oil, for brushing

2% plain Greek yogurt, for serving

1. Make the filling: In a large rondeau (a large straight-sided pan that's a cross between a sauté pan and a cooking pot), combine the bell peppers, zucchini, carrot, and onions. Sprinkle with a little salt (which helps to help draw out the moisture) and cook over medium heat until the vegetables have softened a little and some of the liquid they produce has evaporated, 6 to 10 minutes.

2. Stir in the tomato paste, mixing it in thoroughly, and continue to cook the vegetables until they look slightly softened. Stir in the tomato coulis (for flavor and texture) and cook until the tomato coulis and paste have caramelized and the vegetables are soft and cooked through, another 5 to 10 minutes.

3. Transfer the vegetable mixture to a mesh sieve set over the sink and leave it for about 15 minutes to drain off the excess liquid.

4. Make the eggplant: Preheat the oven to 375°F. Line a baking sheet with parchment paper.

5. Using a sharp knife, cut off the top end of each baby eggplant, halve them lengthwise, and scoop out the flesh, leaving a little flesh near the skin for stability. Place the eggplants, skin side down, on the baking sheet. Brush lightly with olive oil. Bake for 35 to 40 minutes, or until the eggplants are tender. Remove the eggplants from the oven. Reduce the oven heat to 325°F.

6. Coat a large sheet pan with some tomato coulis diluted with water—this is just to help prevent sticking. Place the eggplant halves, skin side down, on the tray. Transfer the vegetable filling to a pastry bag. Fill the eggplant halves with the filling. (Alternatively, you can simply add the filling with a large spoon.)

7. Bake the stuffed eggplants for 35 to 40 minutes, or until the filling looks baked and set. Remove the baking tray from the oven and allow the eggplants to cool for 20 to 30 minutes.

8. Serve the slightly cooled eggplants with a dollop of Greek yogurt on top of each half.

STUFFED ZUCCHINI (ZUCCHINI GEMISTA)

Stuffed vegetables are a great way to pack a lot of flavor into a compact space—this recipe incorporates a number of Pillar Foods, and the dollop of yogurt adds creaminess and rounds out this dish perfectly.

SERVES 8

8 large zucchini

½ cup olive oil

1 bunch scallions (white and light-green parts only), thinly sliced, plus more for garnish

2 garlic cloves, minced

2 cups brown rice

1 cup chopped fresh flat-leaf parsley leaves (no stems)

1 cup chopped fresh dill leaves (no stems)

¼ cup chopped fresh mint leaves (no stems)

Salt and freshly ground black pepper

3 cups vegetable stock or water

Greek yogurt, for garnish

1. Thoroughly wash the zucchini. With the back of a sharp knife, scrape the zucchini to remove any blemishes, but leave on the skin. Cut the zucchini crosswise into 4-inch lengths. Using a melon baller or a vegetable corer, carefully hollow out the zucchini pieces, leaving a half-inch of skin. Chop the removed zucchini flesh. Transfer the cored pieces of zucchini to a large roasting pan. Reserve the chopped flesh in a large bowl.

2. In a medium sauté pan, heat ¼ cup of the olive oil for a minute over very low heat. Add the scallions and garlic and cook them until soft and translucent, about 5 minutes. Increase the heat to medium, add the chopped zucchini, and cook for 5 more minutes.

3. Stir in the rice, parsley, dill, mint, and 2 cups water. Cook the mixture for another 5 to 7 minutes, stirring occasionally, until the rice begins to absorb some of the liquid. Remove the pan from the heat, season the rice mixture with salt and pepper, and allow to cool.

4. Preheat the oven to 375°F.

5. Using a medium-size spoon, stuff the cored zucchini pieces with the rice filling. Be careful not to overstuff the zucchini pieces since the rice will expand as it bakes. Arrange the pieces lying in the roasting pan in a single layer. Leave about 1 inch of space between the zucchini pieces so they will cook evenly.

6. Pour the vegetable stock over the stuffed zucchini. Drizzle with the remaining ¼ cup olive oil. Cover the roasting pan with foil and bake for 45 minutes to 1 hour, or until the rice is tender and the zucchini pieces are soft.

7. For each serving, arrange 2 pieces of stuffed zucchini on a plate. Garnish with a dollop of yogurt and sprinkle with chopped scallions.

ARTICHOKES WITH RICE AND VEGETABLES

This dish reminds me of the beginning of spring, when the first vegetables become available but it's still cold enough out to need a hearty, warm dish. Using wild rice helps up the nutritional value of this recipe, but more important, it gives an extra layer of earthy flavor.

SERVES 8

8 artichokes
Juice of 3 lemons

1 medium red onion, finely chopped

½ cup olive oil

2 cups fresh or frozen peas

3 medium russet (baking) potatoes, peeled and cut into 2-inch chunks

3 carrots, cut crosswise into ½-inch rounds

Salt and freshly ground black pepper

2 cups wild rice

½ cup finely chopped fresh dill leaves (no stems)

1. Prepare the artichokes as described in Step 1 of Artichoke Stew with Vegetables (page 197), using the juice of one of the lemons.

2. In a large pot over medium heat, sauté the onion until softened, 7 to 9 minutes. Pour in the olive oil and cook over medium heat until it is very hot but not smoking. Add the peas, potatoes, and carrots, and sauté the mixture for another 5 minutes.

3. Drain the artichokes and add them to the pot, along with the rest of the lemon juice, 4 cups water, and salt and pepper to taste. Bring to a boil, reduce the heat to a simmer, cover, and cook for 30 minutes.

4. Stir in the wild rice, dill, and another 3½ cups water. Continue to simmer until the wild rice and vegetables are tender, another 20 minutes.

BRAISED CAULIFLOWER (KOUNOUPIDI)

What makes this recipe unique is how we steep the cauliflower in the tomato sauce, infusing it with tremendous amounts of flavor. Eat this alone for a light lunch, or as a side with some souvlaki for a well-balanced meal!

SERVES 3 TO 4

1 white onion, finely chopped

2 celery stalks, thinly sliced

1 carrot, cut crosswise into ¼-inch rounds

4 large tomatoes, grated (on the large holes of a box grater)

3 tablespoons tomato paste

3 tablespoons olive oil

Salt and freshly ground black pepper

3 heads cauliflower, cut into florets

1. Preheat a large saucepan over medium heat until very hot. Add the onion and sauté until golden brown and beginning to soften, 5 to 7 minutes. Stir in the celery and carrot and cook for an additional 5 minutes, stirring to combine.

2. Add the tomatoes, tomato paste, olive oil, and salt and pepper to taste. Continue to cook until the tomatoes are caramelized, an additional 4 to 5 minutes.

3. Stir in 4 cups water, mix well, and bring the mixture to a boil. Add the cauliflower, turn off the heat, and cover the pot. Allow the cauliflower to steep in the hot saucepan until it is tender and flavorful, 15 to 20 minutes. Taste and season with salt and pepper as needed.

Cook's note: If you prefer your cauliflower very soft, cook it over very low heat to desired degrees of doneness rather than just steeping it.

BRAISED GREEN BEANS (FASOLAKIA)

A favorite of my grandmother's, this green bean recipe is perfect as an accompaniment to some simply roasted chicken or fish. You can substitute sugar snap or snow peas without changing the cooking time for an equally delicious rendition of this dish!

SERVES 4 TO 6

1 medium red onion, finely diced

2 garlic cloves, minced

½ cup extra-virgin olive oil

2 cups tomato puree

2 tablespoons tomato paste

1 pound green beans, ends trimmed

1 cup finely chopped fresh flat-leaf parsley leaves (no stems)

3 tablespoons finely chopped fresh mint leaves (no stems)

1 to 2 tablespoons finely chopped fresh dill leaves (no stems), or 1 to 2 teaspoons dried dill

Salt and freshly ground black pepper

Feta cheese, crumbled, for garnish

Greek yogurt, for garnish

1. Heat a large saucepan over medium-high heat for 3 minutes. Add the onion and cook, stirring occasionally, until soft, about 5 minutes. Add the garlic and cook for another minute, stirring frequently. Reduce the heat to medium, add the olive oil, tomato puree, and tomato paste, and cook for another 4 minutes.

2. Place the green beans on top of the other ingredients in the saucepan. Do *not* stir. Cook covered for 10 minutes.

3. Add the parsley, mint, dill, and enough water to just cover the beans. Without stirring, cook the mixture uncovered for 10 additional minutes.

4. Stir or gently shake the saucepan so that all the ingredients are well combined. Season with salt and pepper to taste. Reduce the heat to low, cover the saucepan, and cook until the green beans are tender, another 30 minutes.

5. Serve immediately, garnished with a little crumbled feta or a dollop of Greek yogurt.

MASHED CAULIFLOWER WITH ROASTED GARLIC

A great comfort food alternative to mashed potatoes, this dish pairs perfectly with Spring Stuffed Leg of Lamb (page 250) or Salmon with Fennel and Leeks (page 232).

SERVES 4

3 garlic cloves, peeled

2 teaspoons extra-virgin olive oil

Salt and freshly ground black pepper

1 head cauliflower

¼ cup vegetable stock

¼ cup 2% plain Greek yogurt, plus more for garnish

¼ cup chopped fresh chives (about 10 chives)

1. Preheat the oven to 375°F.

2. Set the garlic on foil, drizzle with the olive oil, and season with some salt and pepper. Wrap the garlic tightly in the foil and roast for 30 minutes, or until soft and caramelized.

3. Meanwhile, wash the cauliflower and cut it into florets. Cut the stalk into pieces, too. In a large pot of boiling water, cook the cauliflower until it is fork-tender, 12 to 15 minutes. Drain.

4. In a food processor or powerful blender, combine the cauliflower, stock, yogurt, and roasted garlic. Puree or blend until the mixture is smooth (see Cook's note). Taste and add salt and pepper as needed.

5. Fold in the chopped chives. Serve immediately, garnished with a dollop of Greek yogurt, if desired.

Cook's note: Feel free to add more vegetable stock for a smoother puree, and adjust the amount of Greek yogurt up or down, to suit your taste.

FASOLAKIA LEMONATA

These lemon-flavored green beans remind me of summers in Greece as a child, when we'd pick the beans right off the pole. The citrus flavor and tender-crisp texture help this dish work perfectly with Fish en Papillote (page 229).

SERVES 4

¼ cup chopped red bell pepper
2 tablespoons chopped fresh dill leaves (no stems)
2 scallions (white and light-green parts only), thinly sliced
1 teaspoon minced garlic
2 tablespoons extra-virgin olive oil
¼ cup fresh lemon juice
Salt and freshly ground black pepper
4 cups green beans, ends trimmed

1. In a medium bowl, combine the bell pepper, dill, scallions, garlic, olive oil, lemon juice, and salt and black pepper to taste. Set aside.

2. In a large pot of salted, boiling water, blanch the beans until they are tender but still retain some crispness, for 4 to 5 minutes.

3. Drain the beans into a large colander and run them under cold water. Leave them in the colander to drain thoroughly. (Alternatively, you can transfer them to a large bowl of ice water for 1 or 2 minutes, and then drain again. This shocks the beans and helps them to retain their bright color.) Transfer the beans to a large serving bowl.

4. Pour the vegetable mixture over the beans and mix well until they are thoroughly coated. Taste, add additional salt and pepper as needed, and toss again.

WILD GREENS IN TOMATO SAUCE (HORTA GIAHNI)

This traditional Cretan side dish is one I often eat as an afternoon snack to keep myself feeling healthy. Make it as described, or forgo the tomato and most of the water for a fresh and verdant Greek stir-fry!

SERVES 5 TO 6

2 scallions (white and light-green parts only), finely chopped
2 leeks (white and light-green parts only), cleaned thoroughly, chopped
¾ cup olive oil
1 pound fresh spinach, washed
1 pound Swiss chard, torn by hand into bite-size pieces
1 pound kale, torn by hand into bite-size pieces
3 zucchini, cut into 2-inch lengths
2 garlic cloves, minced
3 medium tomatoes, grated (on the large holes of a box grater)
Salt and freshly ground black pepper
Lemon wedges, for garnish

1. Preheat a large saucepan over medium-high heat until very hot. Add the scallions and leeks and sauté until softened, about 5 minutes. Pour in the olive oil and, when it's very hot, add the spinach, Swiss chard, kale, zucchini, and garlic. Sauté for 5 minutes.

2. Add the tomatoes, 2 cups water, and salt and pepper to taste. Bring the mixture to a boil, reduce the heat to low, and simmer until the zucchini is tender, 15 to 20 minutes.

3. Serve the greens with the lemon wedges.

SPANAKOPITA TRIANGLES

Favored by the hosts of *Good Morning America,* these light and flaky triangles are an easy and compact version of the classic Greek recipe. Try cutting them in half after baking for a bite-size hors d'oeuvre sure to delight your guests!

MAKES ABOUT 3 DOZEN TRIANGLES

Four 10-ounce bags fresh spinach, stemmed and chopped
¼ pound feta cheese, crumbled
½ cup 2% plain Greek yogurt
1 large onion, pureed
1 bunch fresh dill, stemmed and chopped
1 cup olive oil, plus more for brushing
1 box whole-grain phyllo dough, thawed

1. Preheat the oven to 350°F. Line a baking sheet with parchment paper.

2. In a large bowl, combine the spinach, feta, yogurt, onion puree, dill, and 1 cup olive oil. Mix very well with your hands until all the ingredients are well incorporated. Set aside.

3. Unwrap the phyllo dough and cover it with a clean, damp kitchen towel. Remove 1 sheet of the phyllo and place it horizontally in front of you on a work surface. Using a pastry brush, lightly brush it with olive oil. Top this with another sheet of phyllo, and brush that sheet with some olive oil as well. Using a sharp knife, cut the phyllo into 6 strips (about 12 x 2¾ inches).

4. Place 1 heaping teaspoon of filling near one corner of a strip, and then fold the corner of the strip over to enclose the filling, forming a triangle (the way you would fold a flag). Continue folding, keeping the triangle shape intact. If you have a little phyllo overhang, simply brush it with olive oil and fold it onto itself. Place

your phyllo triangle on the baking sheet and brush the top with more olive oil. Continue making more triangles until you run out of phyllo dough or spinach filling.

5. Bake the spanakopita triangles for 10 to 15 minutes, or until golden brown. Cool slightly before serving.

PUMPKIN AND ZUCCHINI PIE (KOLOKITHOPITA)

In this recipe for a beautiful savory pie perfect for the autumn harvest, pumpkin and zucchini work together with yogurt and *anthotyro* (ricotta cheese) to create a healthy yet indulgent dish, excellent to eat as a meal itself, or as something to pair with Roka Salad (page 173).

SERVES 6 TO 8

One 2-pound pumpkin
Salt and freshly ground black pepper
2 medium zucchini
½ cup milk
4 eggs
2 medium red onions, grated
3 tablespoons olive oil, plus more for the baking pan
¾ cup anthotyro (Greek part-skim ricotta cheese)
½ cup 2% plain Greek yogurt, plus more for garnish
1 cup ground oats (blend old-fashioned or quick-cooking oats in a blender or spice grinder)

1. Rinse the pumpkin and slice off the top and bottom. Using a sharp knife, carefully remove the rind. Cut the pumpkin in half and remove the seeds. Grate the pumpkin on the large holes of a box grater. Place the grated pumpkin in a sieve or colander set in the sink, sprinkle it with salt, and allow it to stand for 30 minutes in order to extract all the excess moisture.

2. Meanwhile, rinse, peel, and grate the zucchini, using the large holes of the box grater. Transfer the zucchini to a separate sieve, and sprinkle it with a pinch of salt. Allow it to stand for 30 minutes in order to remove any excess moisture.

3. Preheat the oven to 350°F. Coat a 9-inch round baking pan with olive oil or line it with a parchment paper round.

4. In a large bowl, combine the milk and eggs. Beat them lightly with a fork or whisk, just to combine. Stir in the onions, zucchini, pumpkin, 3 tablespoons of olive oil, anthotyro, and yogurt. Mix thoroughly to combine. Gradually stir in the ground oats to form a thick batter. Season the batter with some salt and pepper.

5. Transfer the batter to the baking pan. Bake the pie for about 20 minutes, or until golden brown.

6. Remove the pie from the oven and allow it to cool for 15 minutes. Run a small knife around the inside edge of the pan to detach the pie from the pan. Place a serving plate over the pan and invert the pan so that the pie releases onto the serving plate; now transfer it easily onto another serving plate so it is right-side up. Cut the pie into wedges and serve with a dollop of Greek yogurt.

WILD GREENS PIE (HORTOPITA)

I love this pie because it's moist but not soggy, flavorful but not overwhelming, and healthy because it includes many different leafy greens and nutrients.

SERVES 12 TO 24

Salt
4 cups chopped mustard greens
4 cups chopped dandelion greens
4 cups chopped spinach
4 cups chopped kale
4 cups chopped Swiss chard
½ cup olive oil
1 cup finely chopped scallions (white and light-green parts only)
1 shallot, finely chopped
1 cup finely chopped fresh dill leaves (no stems)
1 cup finely chopped fresh flat-leaf parsley leaves (no stems)
Salt and freshly ground black pepper
Olive oil, for the pan and dough
Cornmeal, for the pan
1 package frozen whole-grain phyllo dough, thawed
1 egg, lightly beaten
Greek yogurt, for garnish

1. Place the mustard greens, dandelion greens, spinach, kale, and Swiss chard in your (clean) sink or a big bowl and salt liberally. Rinse them very well under cold running water. Place them in a large bowl of cold water and allow them to sit for 20 minutes. Drain the greens and pat them dry.

2. In a medium pot, heat the olive oil over low heat until very hot. Add the scallions and shallot and cook until tender, about 9 minutes. Stir in the dill, parsley, and salt and pepper to taste, and cook for another 4 minutes. Remove the pot from the heat and allow the mixture to cool.

3. In a large bowl, combine the greens with the cooled herbs. Using your hands, mix thoroughly to combine.

4. Preheat the oven to 400°F.

5. To assemble the pie, coat the bottom of a 9 x 13-inch baking pan with a little olive oil and sprinkle it lightly with cornmeal. Carefully arrange 1 sheet of phyllo in the pan and press it into the corners. Brush some olive oil on the phyllo. Arrange a second sheet of phyllo over the first, and brush with some olive oil. Repeat with a third sheet of phyllo.

6. Transfer the greens to the baking pan and spread evenly over the phyllo. Fold the overhanging phyllo over and onto the filling. Arrange another sheet of phyllo on top of the greens and brush with olive oil. Repeat with 2 more sheets of phyllo. Use a paring knife to remove the overhanging phyllo dough from the sides of the pie. Use the same knife to score the pie into squares or diamonds, just through the top layer of phyllo. Brush with the egg wash.

7. Bake the pie for 20 minutes. Remove it from the oven and lightly sprinkle the top of the pie with a little water, which lends crunchiness to the crust. Return the pie to the oven for another 10 to 15 minutes, or until the phyllo is golden brown. Remove the pie from the oven and allow it to cool for about 20 minutes. Serve the pie hot or cold, with a dollop of Greek yogurt.

CARROT AND HALLOUMI CROQUETTES
(KAROTOPITES ME HALLOUMI)

I love these croquettes because they are well-balanced and tasty, as well as beautiful! The color of the carrots and the brightness of the dressing make this dish dance across your palate. Vary the size of your croquettes depending on what you want them for—they're great for hors d'oeuvres, a light bite, or a beta-carotene–filled lunch!

SERVES 4 TO 6

¼ pound halloumi cheese, roughly chopped, plus ⅓ pound more, cut into ½-inch slices

8 large carrots, coarsely grated or shredded

¼ cup 2% plain Greek yogurt

2 bunches scallions, finely sliced

1 bunch fresh mint, stemmed and chopped

4 eggs, beaten

Salt and freshly ground black pepper

⅔ cup whole-grain or gluten-free flour, for binding

4 tablespoons olive oil, more as needed

1 teaspoon whole-grain mustard

2 tablespoons fresh lemon juice

Chopped fresh flat-leaf parsley leaves (no stems), for garnish

1. In a large bowl, combine the chopped halloumi and the carrots. Stir in the yogurt, scallions, mint, and eggs, and mix thoroughly. Season with salt and pepper. Slowly stir in the flour, a few teaspoons at a time, and mix well until a thick batter forms.

2. Line a large rimmed sheet pan with parchment paper and rub the paper with a little olive oil to prevent sticking. Spread out the batter so that it covers the baking sheet, using a spatula to smooth it evenly. Cover the baking sheet with plastic wrap and refrigerate it for at least 30 minutes.

3. Preheat the oven to 350°F. Line another baking sheet with parchment paper and set aside.

4. Remove the plastic wrap from the chilled, batter-filled baking sheet and bake for about 15 minutes, or until golden and crispy on top. Remove the baking sheet from the oven and allow to cool slightly. Using a sharp knife or a cookie or biscuit cutter, cut out the croquettes until they are about the size of halloumi slices.

5. Arrange the croquettes in a single layer on the second baking sheet. Return to the oven and bake for 5 minutes.

6. Heat a large grill pan over medium heat for about 1 minute. Working in batches, grill the halloumi slices for 2 to 3 minutes per side, until they are softened and grill marks appear.

7. In a small bowl, whisk together the mustard, lemon juice, 4 tablespoons olive oil, and salt and pepper to taste.

8. Arrange the croquettes and the halloumi slices on a large platter, alternating them in rows. Drizzle the mustard-lemon mixture over them, and sprinkle the parsley on top.

ZUCCHINI CROQUETTES (KOLOKITHOKEFTEDES)

These delicate zucchini croquettes make for an excellent canapé, appetizer, or side dish. The flavor of the fresh herbs really comes through, making this great for pairing with any of the dips, especially the Roasted Beet–Yogurt Dip (page 275).

SERVES 10 TO 12

2 large zucchini
Salt and freshly ground black pepper
1 shallot, chopped
3 scallions, finely chopped
¼ bunch fresh mint, stemmed and finely chopped, plus more for garnish
¼ bunch fresh dill, stemmed and finely chopped
¼ bunch fresh basil, stemmed and finely chopped
1 egg, beaten
½ cup crumbled or grated feta cheese
⅓ cup grated Kefalograviera cheese (or a hard grating cheese like Pecorino Romano)
¼ cup ground oats, or more as needed (blend old-fashioned or quick-cooking oats in a blender or food processor until coarsely ground)
Greek yogurt, for serving

1. Preheat the oven to 350°F. Line a baking sheet with parchment paper.

2. Grate the zucchini into a large bowl, using the large holes of a box grater. Sprinkle with some salt and stir well. (The salt will help remove moisture from the zucchini.) Transfer the grated zucchini to a clean kitchen towel, fold up the edges of the towel, and twist both ends of the towel in opposite directions to wring all the excess moisture from the squash.

3. In the same large bowl, combine the zucchini, shallot, scallions, mint, dill, basil, egg, feta, Kefalograviera, and pepper to taste, and mix well. Stir in the oats gradually, until the mixture thickens into a stiff batter.

4. Form croquettes on the baking sheet by scooping out mounds of batter by the heaping tablespoon. Bake the croquettes for 10 to 15 minutes, or until golden brown and soft, but not wet, to the touch. Remove the croquettes from the oven, allow them to rest for 3 minutes, and serve them with yogurt and chopped fresh mint.

TOMATO FRITTERS (DOMATOKEFTEDES)

Tomatoes, basil, and cheese are the basis for many Mediterranean dishes. My take on this classic pairing combines the ingredients in a different way, harnessing all the sweet tomato flavor with the brininess of capers, and topping it with fresh basil and tart Greek yogurt to balance it out.

SERVES 8

4 medium tomatoes

Boiling water

1 medium zucchini

½ medium red onion

1 cup ground oats (blend old-fashioned or quick-cooking oats in a blender or food processor until coarsely ground)

½ cup finely chopped fresh dill

2 tablespoons finely chopped fresh flat-leaf parsley

1 teaspoon capers, rinsed and finely chopped

Salt and freshly ground black pepper

Olive oil, for frying

Fresh basil leaves, for garnish

Greek yogurt, for serving

1. Using a sharp knife, make a small X on the bottom of each tomato. Place the tomatoes in a heatproof medium bowl, cover them with boiling water, and let stand for 1 or 2 minutes. Remove the tomatoes from the water and peel them. The skins should slip off easily. Grate the tomatoes on the large holes of a box grater.

2. Grate the zucchini and onion, also on the large holes of the box grater. Press all the vegetables, including the tomato, in a fine-mesh sieve or squeeze them in a kitchen towel to remove excess liquid.

3. In a large bowl, combine the tomatoes, zucchini, onion, oats, dill, parsley, capers, and salt and pepper to taste. Using your hands, knead the mixture until all the ingredients are well combined. Cover the bowl with plastic wrap and refrigerate for 30 minutes so that the flavors will develop and the batter will set.

4. Preheat the oven to 350°F. Line a baking sheet with parchment paper.

5. Into a large, heavy skillet, pour ½ inch of olive oil. Heat the oil over medium heat until it looks cloudy but is not smoking. Drop large spoonfuls of the batter into the hot oil and fry until the edges are crisp and golden. Flip the fritters, using a large slotted spoon or a spatula, and cook on the other side.

6. When the fritters are evenly golden, transfer them to the baking sheet. Bake for 8 to 10 minutes, or until they are thoroughly cooked. Serve the fritters warm, garnished with basil leaves and a spoonful of yogurt for dipping.

Cook's note: If you like, you may bake the fritters in the oven and avoid frying them at all. Line a baking sheet with parchment paper, brush it with a little olive oil, and form fritters, using a large spoon and making sure they are evenly spaced on the baking sheet. Bake the fritters in a preheated 350°F oven for 15 to 20 minutes, or until golden and crisp on the outside and thoroughly cooked on the inside.

MUSHROOM RISOTTO (KRITHARAKI ME MANITARIA)

This is my modern take on a mushroom risotto—I enjoy using pasta in novel ways, and find that mushrooms give a very unctuous and satisfying flavor to anything cooked with them. Feel free to add some sautéed asparagus to this dish for a crunchy kick!

SERVES 8 TO 10

1 onion, very finely chopped (by hand or in the food processor)
Salt and freshly ground black pepper

1 cup grated tomato (grated on the large holes of a box grater)

2 garlic cloves, minced

2 pounds white button mushrooms, stemmed and cleaned, sliced

1 cinnamon stick

1 bay leaf

1 cup red wine

About 2 cups vegetable stock or water

One 1-pound package Loi Kritharaki Orzo Pasta (or other whole-grain pasta)

Freshly grated Pecorino Romano cheese, for garnish

Fresh basil leaves, for garnish

1. In a large skillet or Dutch oven over medium heat, cook the onion until golden and softened, 8 to 10 minutes, sprinkling it lightly with salt as it cooks. Add the tomato and garlic and continue to cook until well combined.

2. Add the mushrooms and cook until the mushrooms are nicely browned, about 10 minutes. Season the vegetables with salt and pepper, and add the cinnamon stick and bay leaf.

3. Pour in the wine and add 2 cups of stock. Continue to cook over medium heat until the liquid is reduced by one-third. There should be enough liquid in the skillet to comfortably hold all the orzo, about 1 cup. If not, add a little extra water or stock as needed.

4. Preheat a small sauté pan over medium heat for 1 minute. Add the orzo and toast it, stirring, until it turns golden brown and develops a nutty aroma, less than 5 minutes.

5. Carefully add the orzo to the skillet with the mushroom mixture and allow it to cook, stirring occasionally, until it softens, about 5 to 10 minutes. If the orzo has absorbed all of the liquid but isn't quite done, add another ¼ or ½ cup of stock to the skillet. Taste the sauce, and add salt and pepper as needed.

6. Remove the cinnamon stick and bay leaf. To serve, ladle the pasta into large bowls, sprinkle with Pecorino, and garnish with fresh basil leaves.

SPAGHETTI WITH FRESH TOMATO SAUCE

The Italians call it *sugo,* but we Greeks simply call it *domata*—the simplest of pasta sauces made with fresh tomatoes, some herbs and spices, and olive oil. These ingredients come together in a beautiful symphony of flavor sure to delight anyone who eats it.

SERVES 4 TO 6

3 large tomatoes
Boiling water
1 white or Spanish onion, grated
3 tablespoons Greek olive oil
2 garlic cloves, grated or finely minced
1 cup red wine
½ teaspoon hot paprika
Salt and freshly ground black pepper
1 pound Loi Spaghetti (or other whole-grain spaghetti)
Fresh basil leaves, for garnish

1. Fill a bowl with ice and water. Using a paring knife, make a small X on the bottom of each tomato and place them in a heatproof bowl. Pour boiling water over the tomatoes. After 1 to 2 minutes, remove the tomatoes from the water and submerge them in the ice water bath. Peel the tomatoes—the skin should pull away easily. Grate the tomatoes on the large holes of a box grater, or blend them in a food processor.

2. Preheat a large skillet over medium heat for about 5 minutes. Add the onion and sauté until it is softened, 7 to 9 minutes. Stir in the olive oil and when it is very hot, add the garlic. Sauté quickly, just until the garlic is golden, being careful not to let it burn.

3. Add the wine to the pan and cook until it is reduced by about one-fifth. Add the tomatoes, paprika, 2 cups water, and salt and pepper to taste. Boil over medium heat for 10 to 15 minutes to thicken the sauce.

4. Meanwhile, in a pot of boiling, salted water, cook the spaghetti until al dente.

5. Drain the pasta and add it to the pot of tomato sauce, toss to combine, and allow the spaghetti to finish cooking. Transfer the spaghetti to serving plates and garnish with the basil.

TRAHANA

Trahana is an ancient peasant pasta that comes in two varieties, sweet (made with milk) and sour (made with yogurt). Cooked like a porridge and topped with honey, sweet trahana is perfect for breakfast, just like my grandmother used to make. I prefer to use sour trahana, which is different from sweet trahana and pairs beautifully with a sauce worthy of being soaked up to enjoy every last morsel. You can find trahana at a Greek speciality store or order it online.

SERVES 4

2 tablespoons extra-virgin olive oil
Salt and freshly ground black pepper
2 cups sour trahana or cracked wheat or farina (if you can't find trahana)

1. In a large saucepan, bring 3 cups water to a boil. Add the olive oil and a dash of salt and pepper.

2. Add the trahana or cracked wheat and cook over medium-low heat, stirring constantly, until it reaches a porridge-like consistency, 10 to 15 minutes. Season with salt and pepper and remove from the heat.

Cook's note: You can serve this dish with some crumbled feta or a dollop of Greek yogurt for a filling snack, or as the perfect side dish for Grilled Branzino with Tomato-Kalamata Tapenade (page 237).

CANNELLINI BEANS IN WHITE SAUCE (FASOLIA GIAHNI)

My grandmother used to tell me to combat the gas and bloating from beans with lemon juice. Personally, I love this recipe, and while beans can seem heavy, the citrus brightens and lightens the whole thing up—pair them with a crisp Marouli Salad (page 174) for a light lunch!

SERVES 4

1 pound dried cannellini beans
2 medium red onions, finely chopped
1 cup Greek olive oil
1 garlic clove, minced

Salt and freshly ground black pepper

½ cup fresh lemon juice

Finely chopped fresh flat-leaf parsley leaves (no stems), for garnish

1. The night before you plan to serve this dish, place the beans in a large bowl with water to cover by 2 or 3 inches. Set aside to soak overnight.

2. The next day, drain the beans into a colander and discard the soaking liquid. Place the beans in a large pot, add water to cover, bring to a boil and cook until they are fairly soft, about 30 minutes. Remove the beans from the heat and drain them into a large colander, discarding the cooking liquid. Rinse the beans well and drain them again.

3. Meanwhile, in a separate large pot, sauté the onions until golden and softened, 8 to 10 minutes. Stir in the olive oil, garlic, 4 cups water, and salt and pepper to taste. Bring the mixture to a boil.

4. Add the beans to the pot with the onions. Reduce the heat to low and simmer the mixture until the beans are tender and the sauce has thickened, about 30 minutes. Remove the pot from the heat, add the lemon juice, and allow the beans to rest for about 10 minutes so they will absorb some of the cooking liquid. Garnish with parsley.

Cook's note: The cooking time for this dish will vary depending on the quality and origin of the beans, so be sure to check the beans for tenderness and adjust the timing as needed. If necessary, add water so the beans don't dry out.

BLACK-EYED BEANS WITH SPINACH AND SWISS CHARD

One of my favorite places in the United States is Charleston, South Carolina—it's beautiful, full of history, and most important, the food is amazing. I especially love their black-eyed beans, or peas (they are the same thing). This recipe pays homage to my childhood and my first trip to Charleston.

SERVES 4 TO 6

¾ pound dried black-eyed beans (peas)

1 medium red onion, grated

Salt and freshly ground black pepper

¼ cup olive oil

1 carrot, finely chopped

1 pound spinach, roughly chopped

1 pound Swiss chard, roughly chopped

2 medium tomatoes, grated (on the large holes of a box grater)

1. Place the black-eyed beans into a large bowl and add lukewarm water to cover them by 2 or 3 inches. (This will reduce the cooking time.) Set the beans aside for at least 5 hours.

2. In a large pot over medium heat, sauté the onion and a pinch of salt until softened and golden, 7 to 9 minutes. Stir in the olive oil and carrot and sauté until the carrot begins to soften and caramelize, another 3 to 4 minutes.

3. Drain the beans into a colander and discard the soaking water. Add the beans to the pot with the onion, along with the spinach, Swiss chard, tomatoes, 2 cups water, and salt and pepper to taste. Bring to a boil and cook over medium-low heat, stirring occasionally, until the beans are tender and most of the liquid has been absorbed, 15 to 20 minutes. (If the beans start to dry out, add some boiling water to the pot.)

BRAISED GIANT BEANS WITH SPINACH
(GIGANTES ME SPANAKI)

Vegans who have eaten my food know that my braised giant beans are worthy of even the pickiest of eaters. The key to this dish is the cooking time and addition of spinach at the end, making it both extremely healthy and incredibly tasty.

SERVES 6

1 pound dried giant beans (gigantes)

2 medium red onions, finely chopped

¼ cup olive oil

2 medium carrots, sliced into rounds

1 celery stalk, finely chopped

1 bunch fresh parsley, stemmed and finely chopped

1 bunch fresh dill, stemmed and finely chopped

2 garlic cloves, minced

3 cups tomato puree

Salt and freshly ground black pepper

1 pound fresh spinach, washed and stemmed

1. The night before you plan to serve this dish, place the beans in a large bowl with water to cover by 2 or 3 inches. Set aside to soak overnight. (Soaking the beans overnight reduces the cooking time.)

2. The following day, drain the beans, discard the soaking liquid, and place them in a large saucepan. Add enough water to cover the beans by 3 inches. Bring to a boil over medium-high heat and cook until tender, 45 minutes to 1 hour. Drain the beans into a large colander.

3. Preheat the oven to 400°F.

4. Preheat a large saucepan over medium heat for 1 minute. Add the onions and sauté until golden and softened, about 7 to 8 minutes. Stir in the cooked beans and olive oil and continue to cook, stirring occasionally, for about 5 minutes. Add the carrots, celery, parsley, dill, garlic, tomato puree, and salt and pepper to taste. Bring to a boil, then remove the pan from the heat.

5. Transfer the mixture to a medium baking dish. Bake for about 45 minutes, or until the beans are tender.

6. Remove the baking dish from the oven and stir in the spinach. Set the dish aside for about 5 minutes before serving, to allow the flavors to blend.

GREEK SPLIT PEAS (FAVA)

Fava, the most beloved of all bean dishes in the Greek repertoire, can be eaten on its own or—as I do—paired with Crab Cakes (page 231), or even as a dip with some Whole-Grain Pita Chips (page 281). This recipe asks to be played with, so have no fear of doing so and tailoring it to your taste!

SERVES 4

1 pound yellow split peas

2 medium red onions, finely diced or grated

Salt and freshly ground black pepper

3 cups vegetable stock or water

½ teaspoon ground cumin

½ cup Greek olive oil

OPTIONAL GARNISHES

Juice of 1 lemon

½ bunch fresh flat-leaf parsley, stemmed and finely chopped

¼ cup capers (see Cook's note)

1 medium red onion, finely chopped (raw or you can soften it in a pan for 5 minutes)

Greek olive oil, for drizzling

1. Soak the split peas in a bowl of water for 30 minutes. (This will help them cook faster.)

2. In a skillet over medium heat, sauté the onion with a pinch of salt until it is golden brown, 8 to 10 minutes. Remove from the heat and set aside.

3. Drain the split peas and transfer them to a large pot. Add the stock and the onion. Bring the mixture to a boil, reduce the heat to a simmer, and cook until the split peas are soft, about 40 minutes.

4. Add the cumin, olive oil, and salt and pepper to taste. Simmer until the mixture has the consistency of porridge, about 15 minutes. Continue to cook for another 10 minutes, mixing well so that it retains its porridge-like consistency, or remove from the heat and pulse in a blender or food processor until it is mostly smooth.

5. Transfer to bowls and serve with as many garnishes as you like.

Cook's note: If you use capers, first soak them in water for 10 to 15 minutes to reduce their saltiness.

COLD RED LENTIL FAUX MEATBALLS

These faux meatballs, which hail from the Aegean Islands, are extremely flavorful and satisfying, with a wonderful texture that is perfectly matched with the romaine hearts. Eat them for a nourishing lunch or serve as a vegan canapé at your next cocktail party!

SERVES 8 TO 10

1 cup red lentils, rinsed
1 cup bulgur
1 medium red onion, finely chopped
2 tablespoons tomato paste
2 teaspoons ground cumin
½ cup olive oil
1 cup finely chopped fresh flat-leaf parsley leaves (no stems)
Juice of 1 lemon
1 tablespoon paprika
Salt and freshly ground black pepper
Romaine lettuce leaves, for serving
Lemon wedges, for garnish

1. In a medium saucepan, combine the lentils with 3 cups cold water. Bring to a boil, reduce the heat to a simmer, and cook, stirring occasionally, until most of the water has been absorbed, 35 to 45 minutes.

2. Stir in the bulgur and continue to cook until all the water has been absorbed. Remove the saucepan from the heat, cover, and set aside.

3. In a medium skillet over medium heat, sauté the onion until soft, about 10 minutes. Stir in the tomato paste, cumin, and olive oil. Cook over medium heat, stirring, until the tomato paste looks caramelized, about 5 minutes.

4. Transfer the tomato paste mixture to the saucepan with the lentils and bulgur and stir well to combine. Set aside to cool for about 10 minutes.

5. Stir in the parsley, lemon juice, paprika, and salt and pepper to taste. Cover with plastic wrap and refrigerate for 1 hour or until chilled.

6. Using a large spoon, scoop out portions of the mixture, shape into balls (however large you like), and arrange on a large platter. Serve the balls with romaine leaves, garnished with lemon wedges.

POLISPORIA

Eaten after religious fasts, this simple recipe is one of the most nourishing in this book. Beans and whole grains can be dressed as savory or sweet, depending on whether you use lemon or Greek yogurt, or a touch of cinnamon mixed with honey.

SERVES 12

1 cup wheat berries
1 cup dried cannellini beans
1 cup dried black-eyed beans (peas)
1 cup dried yellow split peas
1 cup dried chickpeas
1 cup lentils (any color)
Salt
½ cup fresh or frozen corn kernels
¼ cup olive oil
Fresh lemon juice, cinnamon mixed with honey, olive oil, or Greek yogurt, for serving

1. The night before you plan to serve this, soak the wheat berries, cannellini beans, black-eyed beans, split peas, and chickpeas in separate containers in enough water to cover them each by 2 or 3 inches.

2. The next day, drain the wheat berries and set aside. Drain the cannellini beans, black-eyed beans, split peas, and chickpeas, rinse them, and combine in a large pot. Add water to cover the beans by 2 or 3 inches. Boil over medium heat for 35 to 40 minutes.

3. Drain the beans and return them to the pot. Stir in the wheat berries and lentils, along with salted water to cover them by 1 inch. Boil them over medium heat until al dente but tender, about 1 hour.

4. Stir in the corn, olive oil, and salt to taste. Continue to boil over medium for another 30 minutes or until the contents of the pot thicken.

5. Serve the *polisporia* with some fresh lemon juice, cinnamon mixed with honey, olive oil, or Greek yogurt, according to your personal taste.

KEFTEDES WITH PLIGOURI (BULGAR PATTIES), FRESH HERBS, AND A LEMON VERBENA YOGURT SAUCE

Eating healthy doesn't have to be a chore, and these herbaceous bulgur patties demonstrate how gratifying nourishment can be. The lemon verbena yogurt sauce ties the whole dish together, but feel free to use other herbs in the patties or sauce for different versions of this recipe.

SERVES 8 TO 10

FOR THE BULGUR PATTIES

1½ cups bulgur

2 small zucchini, finely grated

2 tablespoons finely chopped fresh basil leaves (no stems)

2 tablespoons finely chopped fresh flat-leaf parsley leaves (no stems)

2 tablespoons finely chopped fresh mint leaves (no stems)

1 scallion (white and light-green parts only), finely chopped

3 tablespoons olive oil

3 tablespoons anthotyro (Greek ricotta cheese)

3 tablespoons crumbled feta cheese

Salt and freshly ground black pepper

Ground oats, as needed (blend old-fashioned or quick-cooking oats in a blender or food processor until coarse)

FOR THE YOGURT SAUCE

½ cup 2% plain Greek yogurt

¼ cup 2% milk

1 tablespoon fresh lemon juice

2 tablespoons finely chopped lemon verbena

Salt and freshly ground black pepper

Black sesame seeds, for garnish

1. Prepare the bulgur patties: Rinse the bulgur very well in a colander under cold running water. Transfer to a large bowl and add warm water to cover. Set the bowl aside for 5 to 10 minutes, or until the bulgur softens but is still al dente. Drain the bulgur thoroughly.

2. In a large bowl, combine the bulgur, zucchini, basil, parsley, mint, scallion, olive oil, ricotta, feta, and salt and pepper to taste. Mix very well, using your hands. Taste and add extra salt and pepper as needed. If the mixture is very wet and won't come together, stir in a little ground oats.

3. Using your hands, shape the mixture into small patties the size of a hockey puck and place on a large plate. Cover with plastic and refrigerate for 1½ to 2 hours, or until they're solid and firm.

4. Meanwhile, make the yogurt sauce: In a blender or food processor, combine the yogurt, milk, lemon juice, lemon verbena, and salt and pepper to taste. Pulse a few times, until the ingredients are well incorporated, scraping down the sides a few times as needed.

5. To serve, sprinkle the patties with the black sesame seeds, and serve the yogurt sauce on the side.

BARLEY RUSKS WITH TOMATOES (DAKOS ME DOMATES)

I affectionately refer to this dish as the Greek bruschetta—a crunchy whole-grain platform to complement the bright flavor of fresh tomatoes and the sharp, briny character of the feta. You can find barley rusks at a health-food store, Greek specialty stores, or online, but if you strike out, substitute dense, whole-grain bread that has been toasted until crunchy.

SERVES 6 TO 8

¾ cup anthotyro (Greek ricotta cheese)
¾ cup crumbled feta cheese
Salt and freshly ground black pepper
2 very ripe medium tomatoes, grated (on the large holes of a box grater)
½ cup olive oil, plus more for drizzling
Dried oregano
3 tablespoons red wine vinegar
8 small barley rusks

Chopped fresh flat-leaf parsley leaves (no stems), for garnish

Chopped olives, for garnish

1. In a medium bowl, combine the ricotta and feta. Sprinkle it with black pepper to taste.

2. In a second bowl, toss the grated tomatoes with the olive oil and oregano, salt, and pepper to taste.

3. In a third bowl, stir together the vinegar and 2 cups water. Arrange the barley rusks on a large plate, and sprinkle the vinegar mixture over the barley rusks to soften them slightly.

4. Spoon some of the tomato mixture on top of each barley rusk. Top each with a dollop of the cheese mixture. Sprinkle with a little oregano and pepper, and drizzle with a little olive oil. Garnish each rusk with some parsley and chopped olives.

GREEK FRITTATA

Perfect for a weekend brunch with family and friends, this vegetable-filled frittata is easy to make, and is sure to impress. Serve it with a cup of Greek coffee for a great start to the day!

SERVES 4

8 cherry tomatoes, halved

½ red bell pepper, cut into julienne strips

½ yellow bell pepper, cut into julienne strips

½ green bell pepper, cut into julienne strips

1 small zucchini, chopped

½ cup chopped red onion

3 eggs

3 egg whites

½ cup milk (skim, 1%, or 2%)

Salt and freshly ground black pepper

2 tablespoons olive oil, plus more for the baking pan

2 tablespoons crumbled feta cheese

2 tablespoons anthotyro (Greek ricotta cheese)

1 tablespoon chopped fresh mint leaves (no stems)

Greek yogurt, for serving

1. Preheat the oven to 350°F.

2. In a large skillet over medium heat, combine the cherry tomatoes, bell peppers, zucchini, and onion. Sauté until they look softened, about 10 minutes.

3. Meanwhile, in a large bowl, whisk together the whole eggs, egg whites, milk, and salt and pepper to taste until well combined.

4. Transfer the vegetables to a 9-inch round pan or an 8 x 10-inch baking pan coated with olive oil (see Cook's note). Add the feta, ricotta, 2 tablespoons olive oil, and the mint. Pour in the egg/milk mixture and stir briskly to combine all the ingredients.

5. Bake the frittata for about 15 minutes, or until thoroughly cooked. Cut into pieces and serve with a dollop of yogurt.

Cook's note: You may bake the frittata in the skillet in which you sautéed the vegetables, as long as the skillet is ovenproof.

SCRAMBLED EGGS WITH FETA CHEESE (KAYANA)

This recipe was passed down from my cousin's grandmother who lived near Sparta. The simple and tasty combination of tomatoes and feta is quintessentially Greek, and wonderfully healthy.

SERVES 4

3 tomatoes

Boiling water

4 eggs

½ cup crumbled feta cheese

½ cup 2% plain Greek yogurt

½ teaspoon dried oregano

Salt and freshly ground black pepper

3 tablespoons olive oil

1. With a sharp knife, score an X on the bottom of each tomato. Place the tomatoes in a heatproof bowl, pour boiling water over them, and let them stand for 1 to 2 minutes. Submerge them briefly in cold water. Drain and peel the tomatoes (the skins should slip off easily). Halve the tomatoes, remove their seeds, and chop them finely.

2. In a medium, deep skillet, simmer the tomatoes over low heat for 5 to 8 minutes, or until their liquid has evaporated.

3. In a medium bowl, whisk together the eggs, feta, yogurt, oregano, and salt and pepper to taste.

4. Pour the olive oil into the skillet and increase the heat to medium. When the pan is hot, pour in the egg/cheese mixture, stirring so that all ingredients are well combined. Cook over medium heat until the eggs are set, 4 to 5 minutes. Serve hot.

DOLMADAKIA

Voted Best Amuse Bouche by *New York* magazine, my *dolmadakia* are the perfect bite-size treats to start off a traditional Greek meal. You'll need grape leaves in the recipe both to make your dolmadakia and to line the pan you steam them in, but if you roll your dolmadakia smaller, a 1-pound jar will do the trick. Serve them drizzled with Ladolemono Sauce (page 277) or with a dollop of Greek yogurt.

SERVES 20

One or two 1-pound jars grape leaves, rinsed and drained (depending on how big you want your dolmadakia, you may need two jars)

FOR THE FILLING

2 cups Arborio or carnaroli rice

1 bunch scallions, minced

1 leek (white part only), cleaned thoroughly and finely chopped

1 large white onion, minced

1 small bunch fresh mint, stemmed and finely chopped

1 bunch fresh dill, finely chopped

5 tablespoons Greek olive oil

½ teaspoon grated lemon zest

2 tablespoons fresh lemon juice

Salt and freshly ground black pepper

FOR COOKING THE DOLMADAKIA

1 medium white onion, chopped

1 or 2 lemons, sliced into rounds

Grape leaves (you'll have some leftover after rolling the dolmadakia)

1 to 2 cups Greek olive oil (use the higher amount for bigger dolmadakia)

½ to 1 cup fresh lemon juice (use the higher amount for bigger dolmadakia)

½ to 1 cup vegetable broth or water (use the higher amount for bigger dolmadakia)

1. Place the grape leaves in a medium pot and add water to cover. Bring to the boil, reduce the heat to a simmer, and cook until the stem ends of the grape leaves can easily be pierced with a thumbnail, about 10 minutes.

2. Drain the grape leaves and allow them to cool slightly, or run them under cold water so they will cool faster. Remove the end stem pieces from each leaf. Keep the grape leaves covered so they will retain their moisture.

3. To prepare the filling: In a bowl, combine the rice with lukewarm water to cover and soak for 10 minutes. Drain.

4. In a large bowl, combine the drained rice, scallions, leek, onion, mint, dill, olive oil, lemon zest, lemon juice, and salt and pepper to taste. Set the rice mixture aside for about 10 minutes so the flavors can blend.

5. To roll the dolmadakia, arrange the grape leaves, vein side up, on a work surface. Depending on how large you want them to be, place 1 teaspoon or 1 tablespoon of the rice filling at the stem end of each grape leaf. Fold in the two sides of the leaf and roll up to enclose the rice filling. Ideally, the filling will stay in the rolled grape leaves. Repeat until you have used up all the filling and grape leaves.

5. Preheat the oven to 325°F.

6. In a large baking pan (at least 9 x 13 inches, or larger), make a bed of the chopped onion and the lemon slices. Over this, arrange some grape leaves in an overlapping pattern so that they cover the onion and lemon. Arrange the dolmadakia on top of the grape leaves, placing them as close together as possible and stacking them in two layers, if possible.

7. Pour the olive oil, lemon juice, and vegetable broth over the dolmadakia. Arrange another layer of overlapping grape leaves over the dolmadakia. Cover with parchment paper and tightly seal with 3 pieces of foil.

8. Bake the dolmadakia until the grape leaves are soft and cooked through, about 2 hours. Allow them to cool slightly. Dolmadakia may be served hot or cold.

Cook's note: When preparing the vegetables and herbs for the filling, you may either chop or mince everything by hand or combine everything in a food processor and pulse until all ingredients are chopped.

SEAFOOD

FISH EN PAPILLOTE

This simple fish recipe is perfect for balancing the delicate flavors of Greece while incorporating many of the Pillars of the Greek Diet, with the added bonus of a beautiful presentation! Serve this with some simply steamed wild greens and/or some wild rice for a perfectly balanced meal.

SERVES 2

Extra-virgin olive oil
1 lemon, thinly sliced
Two 4-ounce portions white fish fillet (such as branzino, cod, or halibut)
Salt and freshly ground black pepper
½ pint grape tomatoes
1 garlic clove, thinly sliced
3 sprigs of fresh thyme

1. Preheat the oven to 400°F.

2. Line a baking sheet with foil, and drizzle the foil with a little olive oil. Fold a piece of parchment paper in half, center it on top of the foil, and arrange the lemon slices on one half as a bed for the fish fillets.

3. Liberally season the fish fillets with salt and pepper and arrange them in a single layer on the lemon slices. Top the fish with the tomatoes, garlic, and thyme, and drizzle with 5 tablespoons of olive oil.

4. Fold the parchment over the fish. Crimp the longer edges of parchment paper together to seal. Roll the 2 shorter edges of the parchment toward the middle so that the fish is fully enclosed in a parchment package. Rub a little olive oil on the outside of the parchment paper.

5. Bake the fish for 13 to 16 minutes, or until the parchment paper puffs up. Serve the fish in their parchment packages.

STEAMED MUSSELS (MYDIA)

Eaten throughout the Mediterranean, steamed mussels are healthy and satisfying as an appetizer or main course, especially when accompanied by a piece of freshly baked bread to mop up the delicious broth.

SERVES 4 FOR A MAIN COURSE

3 pounds mussels
Salt and freshly ground black pepper
⅓ cup cornmeal
¼ cup minced shallot
1 garlic clove, minced
1 cup white wine
2 tablespoons extra-virgin olive oil
3 tablespoons finely sliced scallion
¼ cup chopped fresh flat-leaf parsley leaves (no stems)
Lemon wedges, for garnish

1. Scrub the mussel shells vigorously under very cold running water. Fill a large bowl with very cold water and add a few ice cubes. Sprinkle in some salt and the cornmeal. Add the mussels, making sure they are completely submerged in the water. Set the bowl of mussels aside for about 1 hour. You may see some tiny bubbles rising to the surface of the water—the mussels are eating the cornmeal.

2. Drain the mussels into a large colander, rinse them under cold running water, and refrigerate on a bed of ice until you are ready to use them.

3. In a medium sauté pan, cook the minced shallot over medium heat until softened and golden, 3 to 4 minutes. Add the garlic and continue to sauté until it is golden, another 30 seconds. Watch carefully so it doesn't burn. Stir in the wine and 1 cup water, reduce the heat, and allow the broth to come to a simmer.

4. Carefully add the mussels. Stir in the olive oil and scallion, cover the pan, and cook until the mussels open, 5 to 6 minutes. With a large slotted spoon, remove the mussels, discarding any that have not opened. Transfer the mussels to a large serving bowl.

5. Increase the heat under the pan to medium-high and continue to cook the broth until it has reduced by one-third, stirring occasionally. Taste the broth and add salt and pepper as desired. Pour the broth over the mussels and sprinkle with the parsley. Serve the mussels with the lemon wedges.

CRAB CAKES (KAVOUROKEFTEDES)

Crab cakes are beloved by all across the globe, but can wind up being heavy due to the binding ingredients. In this recipe, I opt for Greek yogurt instead of mayonnaise, which gives the cakes more flavor and a lighter, fluffier texture.

SERVES 4

½ pound lump crabmeat
½ pound jumbo lump crabmeat
¼ cup minced fresh flat-leaf parsley leaves (no stems), plus more for garnish
1 egg, beaten
Pinch of ground cumin
Salt and freshly ground black pepper
¼ to ½ cup 2% plain Greek yogurt
1 to 2 cups ground oats (blend old-fashioned or quick-cooking oats in a blender or food processor until coarse)
Minced chiles, minced garlic, and whole-grain mustard (optional)
Olive oil, for searing and garnishing
Lemon wedges, for garnish

1. Preheat the oven to 350°F. Line a baking sheet with parchment paper.

2. Drain the crabmeat. Pick through it carefully to make sure there are no shell fragments.

3. In a bowl, combine the crabmeat, parsley, egg, and cumin. Season with salt and pepper. Mix to combine thoroughly. Gradually add ¼ cup yogurt. Add ½ cup of ground oats. Add the minced chiles, minced garlic, and/or whole grain mustard, depending on your personal preference. In order for the crab cakes to hold their shape, the mixture should not be too wet or too dry. If the mixture is too wet, add more ground oats and if it seems a little dry, add more yogurt.

4. When the ideal texture has been reached (the patties should hold together without falling apart or looking mushy), form cakes, using about 2 heaping tablespoons for each and shaping them into patties. Pack them firmly so that they don't break during the cooking process. Place the crab cakes on the baking sheet and refrigerate for at least 30 minutes.

5. Heat a large ovenproof sauté pan over medium heat, adding just enough olive oil to coat the bottom of the pan. When the oil starts to look shiny and hazy, carefully add the crab cakes. Sear them until they have a nice golden brown color, about 2 minutes. Flip the cakes and let them cook for another minute. Place the entire pan in the oven for the crab cakes to finish cooking, about 4 to 5 minutes.

6. Place the crab cakes on a plate, and garnish with a squeeze of lemon juice from a lemon wedge and a drizzle of olive oil. Garnish with minced parsley and additional lemon wedges.

Cook's note: Depending on the flavors you like and want to incorporate, you can add other garnishes, or mix in different options—this recipe is easily adapted to your particular taste!

SALMON WITH FENNEL AND LEEKS

I serve only the freshest wild salmon available—it's so full of flavor, you need very few ingredients to make it stand out on the plate.

SERVES 2

1 leek (all of the white part and ½ of the light-green part), diced
½ fennel bulb, diced
Salt and freshly ground black pepper

3 tablespoons extra-virgin olive oil

1 teaspoon grated lemon zest

Juice from 1 lemon

Two 4-ounce portions salmon fillet, skin removed

1 tablespoon capers, rinsed

Chopped fresh flat-leaf parsley leaves, for garnish

Lemon wedges, for serving

1. Soak the leek and fennel in a bowl of cold, lightly salted water for about 10 minutes. Drain the vegetables into a colander, refill the bowl with water, and repeat until the soaking water is clear. In a medium bowl, toss the leek and fennel with the olive oil, lemon zest, and lemon juice. Set the vegetables aside to marinate for 30 minutes.

2. Heat a medium sauté pan over medium-high heat for 5 minutes or until very hot. Lightly sauté the leek and fennel until they begin to sweat and turn translucent, about 10 minutes. Season with salt and pepper to taste. Set aside.

3. Preheat an oiled grill to medium or preheat a grill pan over medium heat for about 5 minutes. Arrange the salmon skin side down (the side where the skin was before you removed it) on the grill or the grill pan, and grill for 2 to 3 minutes. Using a spatula, flip the salmon carefully, and cook for another 2 to 3 minutes for medium-rare. Grill for another 6 to 7 minutes if you prefer your fish to be well-done.

4. To serve, spoon some fennel and leek mixture onto each serving plate, and top with a portion of the salmon. Season with salt and pepper, garnish with capers and parsley, and serve with lemon wedges.

PSARI MICROLIMANO

The combination of light, flaky fish, sweet tomatoes, verdant dill, sharp scallions, and salty feta is perfectly complemented by the anise-flavored splash of ouzo in this modern interpretation of a classic Greek dish.

SERVES 2

Two 6- to 8-ounce portions white fish fillet (such as sea bass or sole)

1 medium white or Spanish onion, diced

Salt and freshly ground black pepper

10 Caramelized Tomatoes (and Coulis) (page 277)

4 tablespoons chopped fresh dill leaves

1 bunch scallions, finely chopped

½ cup crumbled feta cheese, plus 2 tablespoons for garnish

1 garlic clove, minced

1 green bell pepper, cut into julienne

1 to 2 tablespoons ouzo, Pernod, or anisette, to taste

2 tablespoons olive oil

1. Pick over the fish fillets and remove any tiny pin bones.

2. Heat a medium sauté pan over medium-high heat for 4 to 5 minutes. When it's very hot, add the onion, sprinkle it with a little salt, and cook until it begins to sweat and turn lightly brown. Add the caramelized tomatoes and 2 to 4 tablespoons of their juice, depending on how much you have. Cook the mixture over medium heat for 8 to 10 minutes to develop the flavors.

3. Set aside 1½ teaspoons chopped dill, 1 tablespoon chopped scallions, and 2 tablespoons crumbled feta for garnish.

4. Add the garlic, bell pepper, ouzo, 1 tablespoon of the olive oil, and the remaining dill, scallions, and feta to the pan. Stir well and continue to cook for about 10 minutes, or until the mixture thickens to the consistency of a sauce.

5. In a separate medium sauté pan, heat the remaining 1 tablespoon olive oil over medium heat. When it looks hazy but is not smoking, carefully add the fish fillets. Sauté the fillets until they are opaque, 1 to 2 minutes per side. Spoon on the tomato sauce and cook until the fish is cooked to desired doneness, another 3 to 4 minutes. Season with salt and pepper to taste.

6. Serve the fish garnished with the reserved dill, scallion, and crumbled feta.

QUINOA PILAFAKI WITH SHRIMP, LEMON, AND HERBS

Although quinoa is not a traditional Greek grain, my time spent cooking with it in New York has made me a believer! This protein-rich grain has incredible texture that goes well with many ingredients. In this dish it absorbs the rich flavor of the shrimp, taking this simple dish to the next level.

SERVES 4

¾ to 1 pound shell-on shrimp or 10 to 14 ounces shelled and deveined shrimp

2 tablespoons extra-virgin olive oil, plus more for drizzling

1 small onion, finely chopped

Salt and freshly ground black pepper

1½ cups quinoa

½ teaspoon grated lemon zest

1 tablespoon fresh lemon juice

1½ tablespoons chopped fresh dill leaves (no stems)

1½ tablespoons chopped fresh flat-leaf parsley leaves (no stems)

1. If you have shelled shrimp, proceed to Step 2. For shell-on shrimp, remove the heads (if attached) and set aside. Remove the tails. Peel off the shells and set them aside with the shrimp heads. Using a paring knife, cut a ¼-inch-deep line down the back of each shrimp and remove the vein with the tip of the knife. Rinse the shrimp thoroughly under cold running water. If you aren't using the shrimp right away, refrigerate or arrange on a bed of ice.

2. Heat a large pot over medium heat. Add the reserved shrimp shells and heads to the pot (this step does not apply if you're using shelled shrimp). Add 4 cups water to the pot, then pour in a drizzle of olive oil. Bring the mixture to a boil, reduce to a simmer, and add the shrimp. Cook the mixture until the shrimp turn pink and are opaque throughout, 6 to 7 minutes. Using a slotted spoon, remove the shrimp from the liquid and set them aside. Measure out 2¼ cups of the cooking liquid to use for the quinoa.

3. Heat a medium saucepan over medium heat. Sauté the onion with a pinch of salt until soft and light golden, 3 to 5 minutes. (Salt helps leech moisture from onions, which allows them to soften faster.)

4. Add the quinoa to the saucepan and stir until the quinoa looks toasted, about 1 minute. Add 2 tablespoons of olive oil and stir very well so that all the quinoa is coated. Pour in the reserved shrimp cooking liquid. Increase the heat to medium-high and bring the liquid to a boil. Season lightly with salt and

pepper, cover the pan, and reduce the heat to low. Cook the quinoa until it is tender and translucent, about 15 minutes. Remove the saucepan from the heat and drain off 80 percent of the excess liquid. Cover the saucepan and allow it to stand for 10 minutes.

5. Transfer the quinoa to a serving bowl. Stir in the shrimp, lemon zest, lemon juice, dill, and parsley. Season with salt and pepper, if desired.

Cook's note: Adding quinoa to any recipe is a great way to add texture and protein, but many recipes for quinoa turn out very overcooked because they call for too much liquid. By minimizing the original amount of liquid we cook the quinoa with, we ensure cooked grains with a nice bite.

GRILLED OCTOPUS (HTAPODAKI STIN SCHARA)

The all-time best seller at my restaurants is the grilled octopus. Though it doesn't get beaten against a rock before cooking like we do in Greece, in this recipe, by cooking it low and slow we ensure it is tender and juicy on the inside; by grilling it, we give it the perfect char and slight crispness on the outside. Don't be afraid, it's delicious!

SERVES 4 TO 6

2 pounds octopus tentacles (see Cook's note), thoroughly cleaned
1 cup white wine vinegar
1 cup red wine
10 whole black peppercorns
4 bay leaves
Olive oil, for rubbing on the octopus tentacles
Ladolemono Sauce (page 277)
Chopped fresh chives, for garnish

1. Preheat the oven to 170°F.

2. In a heavy Dutch oven or a brasier (a pot that has a thick bottom, making it ideal for slow cooking and braising), arrange the octopus tentacles. Pour in the vinegar and wine. Stir in the peppercorns and bay leaves.

3. Cover the Dutch oven either with a lid or with foil. Bake for about 6 hours, or until the octopus is tender. Remove from the oven and set aside, covered, for about 30 minutes. Uncover and let the octopus rest for another 15 to 20 minutes.

4. Preheat a large grill pan over medium-high heat. Rub each tentacle with a little olive oil. Working in batches if necessary, grill the tentacles, turning once, until they have grill marks on both sides. Remove them from the grill.

5. Serve the tentacles dressed with the Ladolemono Sauce and sprinkled with chives.

Cook's note: When shopping for the ingredients to make this dish, keep in mind that it all starts with the octopus. The larger the octopus and the bigger the tentacles, the juicier the finished dish will be.

GRILLED BRANZINO WITH
TOMATO-KALAMATA TAPENADE

There's nothing quite so delicious as a perfectly grilled piece of fish, unless of course it's paired with a bright and flavorful condiment and a grain to absorb the natural juices. I love serving this dish with Trahana (page 216), a whole-grain peasant pasta, but you can serve it with quinoa or farro for a bit more texture.

SERVES 4 TO 6

FOR THE TAPENADE
1 shallot, finely minced
½ cup pitted, chopped kalamata olives
1 garlic clove, finely minced
1 to 2 teaspoons red pepper flakes (to taste)
¼ cup extra-virgin olive oil
3 tablespoons fresh lemon juice
2 sprigs of fresh thyme
8 grape tomatoes, minced
½ cup chopped fresh flat-leaf parsley leaves (no stems)

FOR THE BRANZINO

2 pounds branzino fillets (or you may substitute flounder)

Extra-virgin olive oil, for coating the pan

FOR THE TOMATO SALAD

1 pint grape tomatoes

3 tablespoons chopped fresh flat-leaf parsley leaves (no stems)

Chopped parsley and extra-virgin olive oil, for serving

1. Make the tapenade: In a medium bowl, combine the shallot, olives, garlic, red pepper flakes, olive oil, lemon juice, thyme, minced tomatoes, and parsley. Mix well and let it rest at room temperature for 15 minutes. Remove the thyme sprigs. Measure out 2 tablespoons of the tapenade and set aside.

2. Prepare the branzino: Rub the remaining tapenade over the fish fillets, using just enough to cover them. Reserve any tapenade left over for serving with the fish, if you like. Refrigerate the fish fillets for at least 30 minutes and up to 1 hour.

3. Preheat a grill pan over medium heat until very hot. Coat the pan lightly with olive oil. Grill the fish fillets until the fish is cooked through and has developed a nice crust, 4 to 6 minutes per side. Remove the fish fillets from the pan and allow to rest for 3 minutes.

4. Make the tomato salad: Preheat a sauté pan over medium heat. Add some of the reserved tapenade and the grape tomatoes to the pan. Sauté until very warm, 5 to 6 minutes. Stir in the parsley, cook for another minute or two, and remove from the heat.

5. Transfer the warm tomato salad to a large plate. Top with some fish and some of the reserved tapenade, about 1 to 2 teaspoons of the tapenade per serving, although you can use more if desired. Drizzle the fish and the salad with a little extra-virgin olive oil, garnish with some chopped parsley, and serve warm.

SALMON SOUVLAKI

Souvlaki is the ultimate in Greek street food—quick and delicious, full of necessary nutrients, with a great many variations for proteins and produce alike. Serving your souvlaki with pita is optional, and feel free to tailor your souvlaki to your taste, by adding other herbs and spices, or substituting different vegetables or proteins.

EACH VARIATION SERVES 6 TO 8

2 teaspoons grated lemon zest

¼ cup fresh lemon juice

3 tablespoons red wine vinegar

1 tablespoon smoked paprika

2 teaspoons dried oregano

2 garlic cloves, minced

¼ cup extra-virgin olive oil

¼ cup finely chopped fresh flat-leaf parsley leaves (no stems)

Salt and freshly ground black pepper

2 pounds salmon fillets, skin removed, cut into 2-inch cubes

1 red bell pepper

1 cup cherry tomatoes

Whole-grain pita bread (optional)

½ cup crumbled feta cheese (optional)

1. Soak some 10-inch wooden skewers in water to cover for about 1 hour (this prevents them from burning when they're placed on the grill). If you're using metal skewers, skip to step 2.

2. In a large bowl, combine the lemon zest, lemon juice, vinegar, smoked paprika, oregano, garlic, olive oil, parsley, and salt and pepper to taste. Add the salmon and toss to coat with the oil mixture. Cover the bowl and refrigerate it for about 30 minutes.

3. Meanwhile, preheat the broiler. Broil the bell pepper 20 to 30 minutes, turning every 10 minutes, to char evenly. (Alternatively, you may roast the pepper over a flame on the stovetop for 10 to 15 minutes, turning constantly until it is evenly charred.) Place the pepper in a bowl, cover the bowl with plastic wrap, and set it aside for 15 minutes to cool. Once cool, remove the pepper's skin and seeds, and cut into 1½-inch-long strips. Set the pepper strips aside.

4. Preheat a grill to high or preheat a grill pan over high heat. Thread the salmon pieces on the wooden skewers, alternating with the cherry tomatoes. Grill the skewers for 1 to 2 minutes per side for medium-rare. Remove the skewers from the heat and set aside for 3 to 4 minutes.

5. If serving the souvlaki without pita, plate the skewers and garnish with feta and the pepper. If serving the skewers with pita, grill the pitas or warm them in a preheated 325°F oven for 5 to 7 minutes. For each pita, layer some roasted pepper, then some souvlaki (skewers removed) and some feta. Serve hot.

BAKED SHRIMP WITH FETA CHEESE IN TOMATO SAUCE (SAGANAKI SHRIMP)

Greek cuisine is full of pairings unfamiliar to the American palate—this classic combination of sweet shrimp, tangy tomato, and salty, creamy feta will make a convert out of anyone!

SERVES 3 TO 4

12 medium shrimp (preferably shell-on, but can be made with shelled and deveined shrimp)
¼ cup extra-virgin olive oil
1 small red onion, grated
½ cup white wine
2 medium tomatoes, grated (on the large holes of a box grater)
½ cup crumbled feta cheese
¼ cup finely chopped fresh flat-leaf parsley leaves (no stems), plus more for garnish
Salt and freshly ground black pepper

1. Preheat the oven to 350°F.

2. If you're using already shelled shrimp, proceed to Step 3. For shell-on shrimp, remove the legs and shells but leave the heads (if they have them) and tails intact. Using a paring knife, cut a ¼-inch-deep line down the back of each shrimp and remove the vein with the tip of the knife. Rinse the shrimp under cold running water.

3. Heat a large cast-iron skillet over medium heat until it is very hot. When it is very hot, pour in the olive oil. Add the onion and shrimp and sauté until the shrimp begin to turn opaque and pink, 2 to 3 minutes.

4. Reduce the heat to low, add the wine, and cook until it is reduced by half. Stir in the tomatoes, feta, parsley, ½ cup water, and salt and pepper to taste. Increase the heat to medium, and bring to a boil. Transfer the skillet to the oven and bake for 10 minutes, until the sauce thickens.

5. Serve garnished with parsley.

GRILLED CALAMARI (KALAMARI TIS SKARAS)

Calamari is an amazing ingredient. Most commonly, it is found battered and fried, but in Greece, we prefer a simple, unadorned method—marinated and grilled, served with a touch of fresh lemon to showcase its truly exemplary flavor.

SERVES 6

¼ cup extra-virgin olive oil
2 garlic cloves, minced
1 teaspoon dried oregano
1 teaspoon dried mint
1 tablespoon fresh lemon juice
Salt and freshly ground black pepper
1½ pounds whole calamari, thawed if frozen
Lemon wedges or slices, for serving

1. In a large bowl, combine the olive oil, garlic, oregano, mint, lemon juice, and salt and pepper to taste.

2. Add the calamari to the bowl and toss until it is well coated with the oil mixture. Cover the bowl with plastic wrap and refrigerate for at least 30 minutes and up to 1 hour.

3. Preheat a grill to high or preheat a grill pan over high heat until very hot.

4. Remove the calamari from the marinade (discard the marinade). Place the calamari on the grill or grill pan and grill it, turning once, until it turns opaque, about 5 minutes.

5. Remove the calamari from the grill and serve it immediately, with the lemon wedges or slices.

OCTOPUS WITH ORZO

If there were one seafood item that screams "Greek," it would be octopus. This traditional pasta dish highlights the beautiful texture and flavor of this delicious protein in a mild manner, helping less adventurous eaters (and kids) expand their palates.

SERVES 8

4 tomatoes
1 pound octopus, cleaned
1 cup red wine vinegar
2 bay leaves
1 medium red onion, finely chopped
½ cup olive oil
1 carrot, diced
½ cup Mavrodaphne wine (sweet Greek wine)
1 cinnamon stick
1 teaspoon whole allspice berries
Salt and freshly ground black pepper
2 cups Loi Kritharaki Orzo Pasta (or another whole-grain pasta)

1. Fill a bowl with ice and water. Using a paring knife, make a small X on the bottom of each tomato and place them in a heatproof bowl. Pour boiling water over the tomatoes. After 1 to 2 minutes, remove the tomatoes from the water and submerge in the ice water bath. Peel the tomatoes—the skin should pull away easily. Dice and set aside for later use.

2. Rinse the octopus under cold running water. Place it in a large pot and set it over medium heat. Add the vinegar and bay leaves, cover, and cook until the octopus is tender, 35 to 40 minutes. Don't be concerned that the octopus will stick to the pan; it will simmer in its own juices, so there's no need to add extra liquid.

3. Drain the liquid from the octopus and set the octopus aside to cool. When cool enough to handle, cut the octopus into ½- to 1-inch pieces.

4. In the same pot, sauté the onion over medium heat until it is softened, 7 to 9 minutes. Pour in the olive oil and heat it over medium heat for 2 to 3 minutes. Add the octopus and the carrot and cook until the onions

start to caramelize and the carrot begins to soften, 2 to 3 minutes. Pour in the wine and cook over medium-low heat until the liquid is reduced by two-thirds.

5. Stir in the tomatoes, 4 cups water, the cinnamon stick, allspice, and salt and pepper to taste. Bring the mixture to a boil.

6. Stir in the orzo and continue to cook the mixture, stirring occasionally, until the octopus and pasta are cooked to your liking (ideally, soft but slightly al dente), 15 to 20 minutes. If the mixture starts to dry out, add a little additional water. Remove the pot from the heat and let it sit for about 5 minutes for the liquids to absorb. Remove the cinnamon stick.

BAKED SALMON WITH YOGURT SAUCE

This recipe is quick and easy for those constantly on the move, full of the omega-3s and calcium needed for optimum functionality. I love eating this with Marouli Salad (page 174) for an energy-boosting lunch.

SERVES 4

Four 4-ounce portions salmon fillet
4 tablespoons Greek extra-virgin olive oil
Salt and freshly ground black pepper
1 medium tomato
Boiling water
1 cup 2% plain Greek yogurt
1 red bell pepper, diced
2 tablespoons finely chopped fresh dill leaves (no stems)
2 tablespoons fresh lemon juice
Black peppercorns, for garnish (optional)

1. Preheat the oven to 350°F. Line a 9 x 13-inch baking pan with parchment paper.

2. Pat the salmon fillets with paper towels and rub them with a little olive oil (approximately 1 tablespoon per fillet), season them with salt and pepper, and place them in a single layer in the baking pan. Bake the fillets for 10 to 15 minutes for medium-well, flipping them halfway through the cooking time.

3. Meanwhile, with a sharp paring knife, score the tomato by making a small X on the bottom. Place the tomato in a small bowl, cover it with boiling water, and let it stand for 1 to 2 minutes. Drain the tomato and submerge in cold water. Peel the tomato and remove the seeds. Dice the tomato and strain it to remove all the liquid.

4. In a medium bowl, combine the diced tomato, yogurt, bell pepper, dill, lemon juice, and salt and black pepper to taste. Stir well.

5. Serve each portion of salmon topped with a dollop of the yogurt sauce and sprinkle with a few peppercorns.

BULGUR PILAFAKI WITH MUSSELS

The combination of bulgur, mussels, vegetables, and herbs and spices makes this dish a one-pot meal that incorporates half of the Pillar Foods of the Greek Diet. Add your own flavorful twist by using seafood stock in lieu of water in the pot after steaming the mussels if you have it, by increasing the vegetables in the recipe, or by taking the heat up a level with extra chile pepper.

SERVES 3 OR 4

1 pound mussels

3 scallions (white and light-green parts only), finely chopped

¼ cup Greek olive oil

½ green bell pepper, diced

½ red bell pepper, diced

½ orange bell pepper, diced

1 fresh chile pepper (Thai bird's eye chiles are preferred, but use whatever kind you like)

2 garlic cloves, smashed

1 cup dry white wine

2 medium tomatoes, grated (on the large holes of a box grater)

½ cup bulgur

A pinch of freshly ground black pepper

Salt

2 tablespoons finely chopped fresh dill

1. Clean the mussels thoroughly under running water and drain them (see steps 1 and 2 in Steamed Mussels, page 230).

2. In a large shallow pot, combine the mussels with 2 cups water. Bring to a simmer, cover the pot, and let the mussels steam for 5 to 7 minutes, or until most of them have opened. Discard any mussels that do not open; transfer the remaining mussels to a platter. Strain the broth through a sieve into a large measuring cup and add enough water to come to 2 cups.

3. In a separate pot over medium heat, sauté the scallions until they are soft, 5 to 7 minutes. Add the olive oil and heat over medium heat until it is very hot. Add the bell peppers, chile pepper, and garlic and sauté until the garlic is browned and the chile is wilted, 2 to 3 minutes.

4. Pour in the wine and cook, stirring, until it is reduced by two-thirds.

5. Add the tomatoes and the reserved broth from cooking the mussels, and bring to a boil over medium heat. Stir in the bulgur, black pepper, and salt to taste. Reduce the heat to low and simmer, stirring frequently, until the bulgur is fluffy, about 10 minutes.

6. Stir the mussels into the hot liquid and continue to simmer, stirring, until all the liquid is absorbed, about 5 minutes. Stir in the dill.

MEAT AND POULTRY

LAMB SOUVLAKI

Lamb is the most traditional meat associated with Greek food, and souvlaki is the ultimate Greek street-food delicacy. The Greek Diet doesn't promote consistent consumption of red meat, so let this recipe be your special treat for the week.

SERVES 6 TO 8

¼ cup extra-virgin olive oil, plus more for drizzling

½ teaspoon dried oregano, plus more for sprinkling on the skewers

Salt and freshly ground black pepper

2 pounds lamb shoulder, trimmed, cut into 2-inch cubes

1 green bell pepper, cut into 1½-inch squares

1 medium red onion, cut into 1½-inch squares

Whole-grain pita bread (optional)

1. In a medium bowl, combine the olive oil, oregano, and salt and black pepper to taste. Add the lamb, toss to coat with the oil, and marinate for about 1 hour.

2. While the lamb is marinating, soak some 10-inch wooden skewers in water to cover for about 1 hour (this will prevent them from burning on the grill). If you're using metal skewers, skip to step 3.

3. Thread the lamb cubes onto the wooden skewers, alternating with pieces of onion and bell pepper. Leave enough space between each piece to ensure even cooking. Drizzle each skewer lightly with olive oil, and sprinkle with salt, pepper, and oregano.

4. Preheat a grill to high or preheat a grill pan over high heat until it is very hot. Grill the skewers for about 2 minutes per side for medium-rare to medium, or until the lamb reaches the desired degree of doneness. Allow the souvlaki to rest for a few minutes before serving.

5. If serving the souvlaki with pita, grill the pitas or warm them in a preheated 325°F oven for 5 to 7 minutes. Remove the skewers from the meat and vegetables. Serve the pita with the souvlaki, or put the souvlaki inside the pita.

GRILLED CHICKEN BREAST (KOTOPOULO PSITO)

An all-purpose recipe, this yogurt-marinated grilled chicken is perfect for adding to salads, eating with vegetables, or using as a vehicle for sauces. Try it with some Tzatziki (page 271) and Black-Eyed Beans with Spinach and Swiss Chard (page 217) for a delicious meal!

SERVES 8 TO 10

2 cups 2% plain Greek yogurt

½ teaspoon mustard powder

3 pounds boneless, skinless chicken breast

Olive oil, for grilling

Salt and freshly ground black pepper

Dried oregano

Sesame seeds, for garnish

Fresh parsley sprigs, for garnish

1. In a large bowl, whisk together the yogurt and mustard powder. Add the chicken, turning to coat all sides. Cover the bowl, refrigerate, and marinate the chicken for 3 hours, if possible. (The marinade tenderizes and flavors the chicken. If you don't have time to marinate the chicken for 3 hours, let it marinate for at least 30 minutes.)

2. With paper towels or a clean kitchen towel, wipe away as much of the marinade as possible.

3. Preheat a grill pan over high heat for 3 to 4 minutes. Coat the chicken with olive oil. Season the chicken liberally with salt, pepper, and oregano. Grill the chicken for 5 to 6 minutes without turning. Flip the chicken and continue to cook for another 5 to 6 minutes, or until fully cooked and the juices run clear.

4. Remove the chicken from the grill pan and allow it to rest for 4 to 5 minutes so that the juices can redistribute. Serve the chicken garnished with sesame seeds and parsley sprigs.

KEFTEDAKIA

This is the recipe that started my culinary career at the age of seven—I quickly became the chef of the house after my father gave his approval, and haven't stopped cooking since! The Food Network loves this recipe because of the unique flavors and easy method—as do I!

SERVES 6 TO 8

1 large white or Spanish onion

1 large tomato

2 garlic cloves, minced or mashed

1 tablespoon tomato paste

½ cup chopped fresh flat-leaf parsley leaves (no stems)

½ cup chopped fresh mint leaves (no stems)

Leaves from 1 sprig of fresh thyme

½ teaspoon dried oregano

2 eggs

¼ cup olive oil, plus more for drizzling on the meatballs

Salt and freshly ground black pepper

1 cup ground oats (blend old-fashioned or quick-cooking oats in a food processor or blender until coarse)

2 pounds lean ground beef

Greek yogurt, for serving

1. Grate the onion on the largest holes of a box grater. Transfer the onion to a large bowl. Grate the tomato on the same side of the grater and add it to the bowl.

2. Add the garlic, tomato paste, parsley, mint, thyme, oregano, eggs, ¼ cup of olive oil, and salt and pepper to taste. Add ½ cup ground oats, mixing well; add the rest gradually. Add the ground beef and mix it in with 2 forks. Be careful not to overwork the meat so your meatballs will be light and fluffy. Cover the bowl with plastic wrap and refrigerate for 1 hour.

3. Preheat the oven to 350°F. Line a rimmed baking sheet with parchment paper.

4. Using a teaspoon, a tablespoon, or an ice cream scoop, depending on how large you want your meatballs, form meatballs. (Alternatively, you can accurately portion the meatballs by evenly spreading the meat mixture on a 9 x 13-inch rimmed baking sheet. Using a paring knife, slice this into sections—whatever size you'd like the meatballs to be. Remove each uniformly sized portion one at a time, and form into meatballs.) Try not to overhandle the meat mixture, since the less you handle it, the lighter and fluffier the meatballs will be.

6. Transfer the meatballs to the lined baking sheet, drizzle with olive oil, and bake for 15 to 20 minutes, or until browned. Watch them carefully to make sure they don't overbake. Serve the meatballs with yogurt.

Cook's note: You can chop the fresh herbs with a knife, kitchen shears, or herb scissors. Using scissors will enable you to preserve the essential oils in the herbs that can be absorbed by a cutting board when cutting with a knife.

Variation: If you like, mix the beef with pork, veal, lamb, or whatever combination you like. You can customize the ingredients or get creative and add your own special twist.

CHICKEN WITH PEPPERS (KOTOPOULO ME PIPERIES)

Shortly after opening Loi in 2011, I made this recipe on *Good Day New York*. One of the hosts, Greg Kelly, loved it so much, he ate the entire dish before the camera could get a picture of the finished plate—all they could film was him wiping his mouth. What a compliment!

SERVES 6

8 red bell peppers

3 large tomatoes

1 whole chicken (3 pounds), cut into 8 serving pieces

1 garlic clove, minced

1 sprig of fresh oregano

1 cup dry white wine

½ cup olive oil

1 large white or Spanish onion, chopped

Salt and freshly ground black pepper

1 teaspoon paprika

½ cup chopped fresh flat-leaf parsley leaves (no stems)

1 bay leaf

1 cup red wine

6 cups chicken stock

Fresh mint leaves, for garnish (optional)

1. Roast the peppers by placing them over an open flame at medium-high heat on your stovetop. Rotate them consistently using tongs until the entire outside is charred, about 10 to 15 minutes. Place in a bowl, cover with plastic wrap, and allow to steam for 15 minutes. Remove the peppers from the bowl, peel the skin using your hands, remove the seeds, and cut into quarters. Set aside.

2. Fill a bowl with ice and water. Using a paring knife, make a small X on the bottom of each tomato and place them in a heatproof bowl. Pour boiling water over the tomatoes. After 1 to 2 minutes, remove the tomatoes from the water and submerge in the ice water bath. Peel the tomatoes—the skin should pull away easily. Remove the seeds, and set aside.

3. In a medium bowl, combine the chicken pieces, garlic, oregano, and white wine. Cover and marinate in the refrigerator for 2 hours.

4. Drain the chicken, discard the marinade, and pat the chicken dry with paper towels.

5. Heat a large, heavy-bottomed pan with a lid over medium-high heat. Add the oil and working in batches, brown the chicken on all sides, 3 to 4 minutes.

6. Add the onion and salt and pepper to taste to the pan and cook, scraping up the browned bits stuck to the bottom of the pot with a wooden spoon, until the onion is soft, about 5 minutes. Then return the browned chicken to the pan.

7. Preheat the oven to 375°F.

8. Stir in the paprika, roasted peppers, tomatoes, parsley, bay leaf, and red wine. Bring the mixture to a boil, reduce the heat to medium-low, and simmer for 5 to 6 minutes to reduce and slightly thicken the pan juices. Add chicken stock, cover, reduce the heat to low, and simmer, stirring occasionally for 5 minutes.

9. Transfer the pot to the oven and bake it for 1 hour, or until the chicken is very tender. Adjust the seasonings. Serve garnished with fresh mint leaves, if desired.

SPRING STUFFED LEG OF LAMB (BOUTAKI YEMISTO)

A celebratory dish in Greece, this stuffed leg of lamb is most commonly eaten after Lent, on Easter Sunday. The light and savory filling marries perfectly with the robust, slightly gamey flavor of the lamb for a beautiful spring meal.

SERVES 8 TO 10

FOR THE MARINADE AND LAMB
4 cups 2% plain Greek yogurt
2 tablespoons whole-grain mustard
Leaves from 3 sprigs of fresh thyme
3 garlic cloves, minced
One 4- to 5-pound deboned leg of lamb

FOR THE FILLING/COMPLEMENT
1 standard size (250g) package halloumi cheese
3 large leeks (white and light-green parts only), cleaned thoroughly and chopped

3 bunches scallions (white and light-green parts only), sliced

1 fennel bulb, diced

Salt

Olive oil

½ pound feta cheese, crumbled

Salt and freshly ground black pepper

1 pound baby spinach

1 to 2 cups 2% plain Greek yogurt

Mustard powder

Chopped fresh flat-leaf parsley or sliced scallions, for garnish

1. The night before you plan to serve this dish, marinate the lamb: In a medium bowl, whisk together the yogurt, mustard, thyme, and garlic. Place the lamb in a large container, pour in the marinade, and turn the lamb so that it is coated on all sides. Tightly cover the container and marinate overnight in the refrigerator.

2. The next day, use paper towels to wipe the marinade off the lamb. Return the lamb to the refrigerator while you make the filling.

3. Make the filling: Grate half of the halloumi on the large holes of a box grater and set aside.

4. Cut the remaining halloumi into ½-inch-thick slices. Heat a grill pan over medium heat. Grill the cheese slices just long enough for them to develop grill marks on both sides. When the grilled halloumi is cool, chop it coarsely and set it aside.

5. Preheat a large sauté pan over medium heat for 3 to 4 minutes, or until very hot. Add the leeks, scallions, and fennel. Sprinkle with a little salt and allow the vegetables to sweat, without any olive oil. When they are translucent, add a touch of olive oil along with both the grated and chopped grilled halloumi and continue cooking until the halloumi starts to melt, a few more minutes. Add the feta and allow the mixture to continue cooking so the flavors marry, 5 to 7 minutes. Season with salt and pepper as needed. Remove the pan from the heat and add the spinach, mixing it into the pan so that it wilts and cooks from the residual heat.

6. Transfer 2 heaping tablespoons of the vegetable mixture to a bowl and set the rest aside for serving later. Slowly add some of the yogurt, starting with ½ cup, and continue adding yogurt until a balanced consistency is reached (1 cup should be more than sufficient, but if you like, you can add more according to your personal preference; but save the remaining yogurt for serving).

7. Preheat the oven to 400°F.

8. Remove the lamb from the refrigerator and place it, deboned side up, on a large cutting board with enough space to stuff and roll it. Place 2 or 3 large spoonfuls of the filling inside the leg of lamb and spread across the length of the leg. Roll up the roast and tie it off with kitchen string so that it will not fall open while roasting, being sure to seal in the filling as much as possible. Place the leg in a large roasting pan and rub the outside with olive oil, and season to taste with salt, pepper, and mustard powder.

9. Roast the lamb for 30 minutes. Reduce the oven temperature to 325°F. Cook, basting the lamb every 20 minutes with the pan drippings, for 35 to 40 minutes, or until it is rare to medium-rare. The temperature of the lamb will be about 140°F. Remove the lamb from the oven and allow it to rest for at least 30 minutes. Slice the lamb crosswise into ½-inch-thick slices that contain meat and filling.

10. To serve, reheat the leek/scallion/cheese mixture quickly over low heat. Transfer it to a bowl and stir in some of the remaining yogurt until the desired consistency is reached. It should be runny, and not too chunky. To serve, plate three slices of the stuffed lamb with a generous serving of the vegetable-yogurt mixture. Garnish the plate with parsley.

CHICKEN WITH DILL

Dill is commonly associated with seafood dishes, but I love this simple chicken recipe because this beautiful herb is the star. Serve this dish for dinner with a small wedge of Spanakopita Triangles (page 206) and some Trahana (page 216) to create a delicious, well-balanced meal.

SERVES 6 TO 8

1 whole chicken (3 pounds), cut into 8 serving pieces
Salt and freshly ground black pepper
1 large red onion, finely chopped
½ cup Greek olive oil
4 small or 2 large bunches fresh dill, stemmed and chopped
3 tablespoons fresh lemon juice (about 1 lemon)

1. Rinse and drain the chicken. Sprinkle it with salt and pepper. Set it aside.

2. Preheat a 12-inch sauté pan or saucepan over medium heat for 5 to 6 minutes. Add the onion and sauté until it is softened, 8 to 10 minutes. Pour in the olive oil. When it is very hot, add the chicken pieces and cook over medium heat, until evenly browned, 5 to 7 minutes, turning to brown on both sides.

3. Pour in enough water to cover the chicken and simmer until the chicken is cooked through, 15 to 20 minutes, stirring in the dill halfway through the cooking time.

4. Remove the saucepan from the heat, add the lemon juice, and move the saucepan clockwise to mix. You want to add the lemon as a finishing touch but not cook it, since heating it will change its flavor.

5. Season the chicken with more salt and pepper as needed.

LAMB FRICASSEE (ARNAKI FRIKASE)

Greeks and lamb go together like peas and carrots, as they say in America. This dish showcases the robust flavors of my heritage in a reserved and elegant way, all brought together in the end by my Avgolemono Sauce.

SERVES 6 TO 8

2 pounds deboned lamb shoulder or leg of lamb, cut into 1- to 2-inch pieces
1 medium white onion, diced
Pinch of coarse salt
3 bunches scallions (white and light-green parts only), chopped
¼ cup olive oil
2 cups vegetable stock or water
½ bunch fresh dill, stemmed and chopped
Salt and freshly ground black pepper
3 heads romaine lettuce, cleaned
Egg-Lemon (Avgolemono) Sauce (page 276)
Leaves from 5 sprigs of fresh mint, chopped

1. Preheat a large pot over medium-high heat until very hot. (You will be browning the lamb to seal in the juices and add a depth of flavor, but since lamb is a fattier type of meat, no oil is needed for browning.)

2. Add the lamb to the pot and sear it on all sides, until nicely browned and beginning to caramelize, about several minutes per side. Remove the lamb from the pot, reduce the heat, and add the onion and coarse salt. (The salt helps leech the moisture out of the onion.) After browning the lamb, there should be little bits of *fond*, the browned bits and caramelized drippings stuck to the bottom of the pan after sautéing or roasting. The fond helps to build flavor in the dish, so as the onion begins to release moisture, use a wooden spoon to scrape up those browned bits and mix them in with the onion. Continue to cook the onion until softened and beginning to color, 5 to 7 minutes.

3. Stir in the scallions. Continue to cook until the scallions lose their bright color and appear softened. Add the olive oil to the pot. Return the lamb to the pot, along with 1 cup vegetable stock and the dill. Season lightly with salt and pepper, cover, and cook over low heat, stirring occasionally, until the lamb is soft and tender, about 1 hour.

4. Using your hands, tear the romaine lettuce into 1- to 2-inch pieces. Add some of the romaine to the pot. Cover the pot again, and allow the romaine to steam for 10 to 15 minutes. Remove the cover and add as much more romaine as will fit into the pot. Cook for another 10 to 15 minutes. Repeat this process until you've used all the romaine. Allow the mixture to cook for another 10 to 15 minutes on very low heat. If it becomes dry, just add a little more stock.

5. Meanwhile, prepare the Avgolemono Sauce.

6. Pour the Avgolemono Sauce gently over the fricassee, mixing well to combine. Season with salt and pepper to taste. Mix in the mint, reserving a little for garnish. To serve, ladle the fricassee into wide-rimmed bowls or plates, and sprinkle with fresh mint.

CHICKEN AND MUSHROOM SOUVLAKI

This hearty version of souvlaki is separate from the others because unlike the lamb or salmon, chicken must be completely cooked through. Serve it with Tzatziki (page 271) and some Couscous Salad (page 175) for a true Mediterranean treat. You can tailor this recipe to your personal taste, adding more vegetables or a different protein, depending on your preference.

SERVES 4

½ cup Greek olive oil
Juice of 2 lemons

1 teaspoon dried oregano

Salt and freshly ground black pepper

2 boneless, skinless chicken breasts, cut into bite-size pieces

8 white button mushrooms, cleaned and stemmed

2 green bell peppers, cut into bite-size pieces

2 medium red onions, peeled and each cut into sixths

Finely chopped fresh dill, for garnish

1. Soak some 10-inch wooden skewers in water to cover for about 1 hour. (This will prevent them from burning when placed on the grill.) If you're using metal skewers, skip to step 2.

2. In a large bowl, combine the olive oil, lemon juice, oregano, and salt and pepper to taste. Stir well to combine. Add the chicken, mushroom caps, bell pepper, and onion. Cover the bowl with plastic wrap and refrigerate for about 30 minutes.

3. Preheat an oiled grill or a grill pan over medium-high heat.

4. Remove the chicken from the marinade and assemble the souvlaki as follows: Thread 1 mushroom cap onto a skewer. Then alternate a piece of pepper, a piece of chicken, and a piece of onion, continuing until the skewer is almost full. Thread another mushroom cap at the end of the skewer. Continue until you run out of ingredients and/or skewers.

5. Grill the souvlaki on all sides, turning occasionally, until the chicken is cooked thoroughly, beautifully browned, and lightly charred with grill marks, 10 to 15 minutes.

Cook's note: If you would like to control how well-done your vegetables are, you can cook them on separate skewers for different lengths of time. But you need to marinate the chicken and vegetables in separate bowls so that you don't cross-contaminate the vegetables with the chicken.

MEDITERRANEAN CHICKEN STEW

Hearty and comforting, this stew can be found with slight variations all over the Mediterranean. I love this version because you can really taste how all the ingredients come together to create a unified, one-pot meal. If you like, serve with some crusty Multigrain Bread (page 282).

SERVES 8 TO 10

1 tablespoon tomato paste
4 cups chicken stock, vegetable stock, or water
1 whole chicken (3 pounds), cut into eight pieces
3 medium eggplants, diced into 1-inch cubes
2 green bell peppers, roughly chopped
2 red bell peppers, roughly chopped
2 garlic cloves, minced
4 medium tomatoes, diced
1 bunch fresh flat-leaf parsley, stemmed and chopped
½ cup olive oil
Salt and freshly ground black pepper
Greek yogurt, for serving

1. Preheat the oven to 375°F.

2. In a medium bowl, dissolve the tomato paste in the chicken stock.

3. In a large baking pan, combine the chicken, eggplant, bell peppers, garlic, tomatoes, parsley, olive oil, and salt and pepper to taste.

4. Pour the tomato paste mixture over the chicken and vegetables. Cover and bake for 30 minutes. Uncover and bake until the chicken is thoroughly cooked and golden, another 30 minutes.

5. Serve with yogurt.

DESSERTS

ROUND BAKLAVA (KYKLOS BAKLAVA)

Perhaps the most famous of all desserts, baklava is synonymous with all things Mediterranean. You can trace the origins back to *gastrin,* a precursor to baklava, in ancient Greece.

MAKES 40

1 cup blanched almonds

2 cups walnuts

½ cup sugar

2 teaspoons ground cinnamon

Greek olive oil

Sesame oil (light or dark)

One 1-pound package frozen phyllo dough, thawed

FOR THE SYRUP

1 cup sugar

1 cup Greek honey

3 whole cloves

1 cinnamon stick

1. In a food processor, roughly chop the almonds and transfer to a large bowl. Lightly chop the walnuts or crush them with the side of a knife and add them to the almonds. Stir in the sugar and cinnamon.

2. In a small bowl, mix together equal parts of Greek olive oil and sesame oil. Have a pastry brush ready.

3. Preheat the oven to 350°F.

4. On a work surface, lay out 2 sheets of phyllo dough. Place 1 on top of the other. Using the pastry brush, lightly brush the top of the sheets with the oil mixture. Sprinkle with some of the nut mixture. Arrange 2 sheets of phyllo on top and lightly brush with the oil. Continue to layer the oil-brushed phyllo sheets with the filling 4 or 5 more times.

5. Top this layered phyllo pastry with 2 more sheets of phyllo, brushing each with some of the oil.

6. Separately, brush 3 sheets of phyllo with oil and stack them on top of one another. Roll the layered nuts and phyllo pastry up in the 3 sheets of phyllo, enclosing the pastry completely, to help make it firm enough to slice. Using a sharp knife, slice the roll crosswise on an angle into small rounds.

7. Line a large baking sheet with parchment paper. Lay the pieces of baklava on the baking sheet, leaving about 1 inch of space between them. If necessary, use a second baking sheet so that the baklava will all fit in a single layer.

8. Brush the tops of each piece of baklava with some of the oil mixture. Bake for 10 to 15 minutes, or until golden brown. Remove the baklava from the oven and allow it to cool on the baking sheet.

9. Meanwhile, prepare the syrup: In a small saucepan, whisk together 2 cups water, the sugar, honey, cloves, and cinnamon stick over low heat. When the mixture simmers, continue to cook until the sugar dissolves and the syrup tastes spicy, about 5 minutes.

10. Pour the syrup over the cooled baklava and let the baklava rest for about 1 hour to soak up the syrup.

Cook's note: Be sure to keep the phyllo dough covered with a clean damp kitchen towel as you work so that it will not dry out. And keep in mind that the amounts for the nuts, cinnamon, and sugar listed in the recipe are guidelines. Tailor the baklava to your taste.

PEARS WITH MAVRODAPHNE SAUCE
(PEARS WITH SWEET RED WINE SAUCE)

These poached pears hail from the ancient days, but you can modernize them by changing what you poach them in! Slice and add them to your morning oatmeal or yogurt bowl, or serve them as a classic dessert.

SERVES 4 TO 8

4 pears, peeled, but with the stems left on
2 cups Mavrodaphne wine (see Cook's note)
1 cinnamon stick

½ cup packed light brown sugar or 2 tablespoons honey

½ cup walnuts

Greek yogurt, for serving

1. In a medium saucepan, arrange the pears in a single layer, stem side up. Add the wine, cinnamon stick, brown sugar, and walnuts, and bring to a boil over medium-low heat.

2. Reduce the heat to low and simmer until the wine sauce is foamy and the pears are tender, 10 to 15 minutes.

3. To serve, place some yogurt in each dish, add either a whole or a half pear, and top with some of the sauce. If you like, remove the cinnamon stick but this isn't necessary.

Cook's note: If you can't find Mavrodaphne wine, try using another sweet red wine like Manischewitz Medium Dry Concord or Port. If you want to be adventurous, try poaching the pears in a sweet white wine, or even some cider or mead! In addition, you may substitute apples for the pears in this dish.

RICE PUDDING (RIZOGALO)

Warm and comforting, or cold and creamy, my rice pudding will make you feel like a kid all over again. Eat it for dessert after a vegetable-heavy dinner (such as Vegetable Stew [Turlu], page 193), or as an afternoon snack with some pomegranate seeds.

SERVES 6 TO 8

1 cup wild rice

1 cup sugar

6 cups 2% milk

¼ cup cornstarch

2 teaspoons vanilla extract

Ground cinnamon, for garnish

Pomegranate seeds, for garnish

1. In a large pot, bring 4 cups water to a boil. Stir in the wild rice. Simmer over low heat, stirring frequently, until the rice is tender and all the water has been absorbed, about 30 minutes, until the rice is tender and all the water has been absorbed.

2. Meanwhile, in a large bowl, combine the sugar and 5 cups of the milk. In a small bowl, dissolve the cornstarch in the remaining 1 cup milk.

3. While stirring with a large wooden spoon, pour the sugar-milk mixture into the pot with the rice and continue stirring, until the mixture come to a boil. Add the cornstarch mixture to the pot and cook over low heat until the mixture thickens.

4. Remove the pot from the heat and stir in the vanilla. Serve the *rizogalo* hot or cold, garnished with ground cinnamon or pomegranate seeds.

ALMOND COOKIES (AMIGDALOTA)

The Greek answer to the macaroon, these light almond cookies are great for satisfying that nagging sweet tooth without overdoing it on the sugar.

MAKES 2 TO 3 DOZEN COOKIES

2 pounds blanched whole almonds
½ pound (1½ cups) confectioners' sugar
2 eggs
2 egg yolks
1 teaspoon rosewater

1. Preheat the oven to 400°F. Line a large baking sheet with parchment paper.

2. In a food processor, pulse the almonds just until they are finely chopped. Watch carefully so you don't pulse them into a powder since this will make the dough hard to handle.

3. In a large bowl, combine the chopped almonds, confectioners' sugar, whole eggs, egg yolks, and rosewater. With your hands, knead to form a firm dough.

4. Mold golfball-size pieces of dough into almond-shaped cookies. Arrange the cookies on the prepared baking sheet, leaving 1 inch of space between each.

5. Bake the cookies for 15 to 20 minutes, or until they are slightly browned and firm on the outside. Allow the cookies to cool thoroughly on the baking sheet. Leaving them to cool on the baking sheets will ensure that they don't break as you remove them. Store the cookies, covered, at room temperature.

LEMON–OLIVE OIL CAKE

This cake highlights the fruit-forward qualities of the olive oil, while balancing out the citrus notes from the lemon. You can substitute a different citrus fruit, or even add some fresh herbs to make this cake yours—I love adding some fresh lemon thyme and serving it with a dollop of yogurt.

SERVES 16

1 cup extra-virgin olive oil, plus more for the cake pan

2 cups cake flour (not self-rising)

3 tablespoons grated lemon zest

4 eggs, separated, plus 1 more egg yolk

¾ cup plus 1½ tablespoons sugar

3 tablespoons fresh lemon juice

½ teaspoon salt

1. Preheat the oven to 350°F. Coat a 9-inch springform pan with a little olive oil. Cut a round of parchment paper to fit the pan, place it on the bottom of the pan, and coat it liberally with some olive oil.

2. In a small bowl, whisk together the flour and lemon zest. Set aside.

3. In a medium bowl, with an electric mixer or an egg beater, beat the 5 egg yolks and ½ cup of the sugar on high speed until the mixture is thick and pale, 3 to 4 minutes. Reduce the speed of the mixer/beater to medium-low and slowly add the 1 cup olive oil and the lemon juice, mixing them until just combined. The batter might look as if it has separated, but that's okay! Using a wooden spoon, mix in the flour mixture just until combined. You don't need the electric mixer for this step.

4. In another bowl, with the electric mixer or the egg beater, beat the 4 egg whites with the salt at medium to high speed until foamy. Continue to beat as you slowly add the ¼ cup sugar, and keep beating until soft peaks form, 3 to 4 minutes.

5. Carefully fold about one-third of the beaten egg whites into the batter and then gently but thoroughly fold in the rest of the egg whites.

6. Transfer the batter to the prepared cake pan and gently rap the pan against a hard surface to release any air bubbles that may have formed during the mixing process. Sprinkle the top of the cake with the remaining 1½ tablespoons sugar.

7. Bake the cake for about 45 minutes, or until it has risen, is a beautiful shade of gold, and a toothpick inserted into the center of the cake comes out clean, with no traces of uncooked batter.

8. Allow the cake to cool in the pan on a rack for 10 to 15 minutes. Run a knife around the inside edge of the pan and release the springform sides. Let the cake cool and rest for another hour. Flip the cake over onto a plate. Remove the bottom of the pan and the parchment paper.

PRESERVED CHERRIES IN SYRUP
(GLIKO TOU KOUTALIOU KERASI)

This is my favorite version of a traditional Greek spoon dessert, which is so called because you eat just a spoonful at a time. The amount of sugar you consume in it is actually quite small. Try it with some Greek yogurt for a classic Hellenic dessert!

SERVES 25 TO 30

1 cup (½ pound) granulated sugar

3 tablespoons honey

2 cups pitted cherries

1 teaspoon grated lemon zest

1 teaspoon fresh lemon juice

1 cup whole roasted blanched almonds or any almonds available

Greek yogurt, for serving

1. The night before you plan to serve this, in a saucepan, combine the sugar, honey, and 1 cup water. Bring the mixture to a boil over medium heat. Add the cherries, stir well, and boil over medium heat until the cherries soften and the liquid becomes syrupy, 10 to 15 minutes.

2. Remove the saucepan from the heat and refrigerate it overnight.

3. The following day, stir in the lemon zest, lemon juice, and almonds. Bring the mixture to a boil over medium heat. Boil until the syrup has thickened, 10 to 15 minutes.

4. Transfer the dessert to clean glass jars, cover, and refrigerate for up to 2 weeks.

5. Serve the *gliko tou koutaliou kerasi* with some yogurt.

Cook's note: Since the preserved cherries have no chemical preservatives, they should always be kept in the refrigerator.

FROZEN GREEK YOGURT

The world is obsessed with Greek yogurt, and for good reason: It's delicious, healthy, and full of protein! I created this frozen version to be made without an ice cream maker, so that everyone can create and enjoy this amazing frozen treat at home!

SERVES 4

2 cups 2% plain Greek yogurt

FLAVORINGS (CHOOSE ONE)
½ to 1 cup fresh fruit (blueberries, blackberries, strawberries, raspberries, peaches, mango, and/or cherries), to taste, plus more for garnish
2 tablespoons Greek coffee blended with 2 tablespoons Greek honey

1. If using homemade yogurt, follow the recipe, but drain for an additional 3 to 4 hours in the refrigerator or in the kitchen, if it's not too warm, in order to remove as much liquid as possible. This helps ensure that the yogurt will have fewer ice crystals when frozen.

2. Put the yogurt in a shallow metal pan and place it in the freezer for 1½ to 2 hours, covered, if you wish. If you're planning on flavoring the yogurt with fruit, freeze the fruit in a separate container for 1 to 1½ hours.

3. Scrape the frozen yogurt into a food processor. If you are flavoring with fruit, add it now and blend until the fruit and yogurt are just combined. The mixture will look a little icy and not especially creamy, but this is fine,

as you will be repeating the process. If you are flavoring the yogurt with coffee, add the coffee/honey mixture to the food processor in place of the fruit. Blend until the yogurt, coffee, and honey are well combined.

4. Transfer the mixture back to the shallow metal pan and freeze for another 1½ to 2 hours.

5. Scrape and spoon the frozen yogurt mixture back into the food processor, blending it until it looks creamier than the first time.

6. Repeat for a third time. When you transfer the frozen yogurt mixture to the food processor this time, blend it until it is smooth and creamy.

7. Store the frozen yogurt in the freezer for 1 to 2 weeks. Serve garnished with the same type of fruit that is in the yogurt, or with a drizzle of Greek honey.

GREEK BAKED APPLES

Wonderful for the fall, these baked apples are my ode to the Big Apple! Served warm with a dollop of Greek yogurt or chilled with a hot cup of tea, these apples are a satisfying sweet treat with a fiber kick.

SERVES 6

½ cup raisins (dark or golden)
Apple juice
6 firm apples, such as Granny Smith, Pink Lady, Honeycrisp, or Braeburn (see Cook's note)
1 cup walnuts, roughly chopped
½ cup almonds, roughly chopped
2 teaspoons ground cinnamon, plus more for garnish
¼ teaspoon ground cloves
½ cup honey, warmed
½ cup Greek yogurt, for serving

1. The night before you plan to serve the apples, place the raisins in a small bowl, add apple juice to cover them by about 2 inches, cover, and set aside.

2. The following day, use an apple corer to remove the cores from the apples. Don't cut all the way through the core, though, as you will be stuffing them. Wash and dry them. Peel them if you like, and set aside.

3. Preheat the oven to 350°F. Line the bottom of a baking dish with parchment paper.

4. In a medium bowl, combine the walnuts, almonds, cinnamon, cloves, and 2 tablespoons honey. Fill the hollowed-out center of each apple with some of the nut mixture. Arrange the apples in the baking dish. Pour the remaining honey over the apples.

5. Bake the apples for 25 to 30 minutes, until they have softened and cooked through.

6. Drain the raisins. Combine the raisins with the yogurt. To serve, place an apple on a serving dish. Top with a dollop of yogurt and sprinkle with some cinnamon.

Cook's note: You may leave on the apple skin or peel it—it's your choice! Firmer apples are better candidates for leaving the skin on. Softer apples are more likely to lose their shape and crumble from the steam if not peeled.

HONEY PIE (MELOPITA)

Melopita translates as "honey pie," but this dish is my healthy version of a ricotta-style cheesecake. Light and fresh with a hint of lemon, this cake has the perfect tang from the yogurt. Serve this with Pears with Mavrodaphne Sauce (page 258) for a decadent dessert, or drizzle with some honey to keep it classic.

SERVES 16

Olive oil, for the pan
1 pound anthotyro (ricotta cheese)
1 cup 2% plain Greek yogurt
3 eggs, lightly beaten
½ cup Greek honey, plus more for garnish
Grated zest of 1 lemon
3 tablespoons all-purpose flour
¼ cup sugar
Ground cinnamon, for garnish

1. Preheat the oven to 350°F. Coat a 9-inch springform pan with olive oil, line it with a round of parchment paper, and lightly oil the paper.

2. In a large bowl, combine the ricotta, yogurt, eggs, ½ cup honey, lemon zest, flour, and sugar. Beat thoroughly, either with an electric mixer or a whisk.

3. Pour the batter into the pan and gently rap it against a hard surface to release any air bubbles.

4. Bake the melopita for 15 to 20 minutes, or until the filling sets. Remove the cake from the oven and let cool. Refrigerate the cake for 2 or 3 hours.

5. Run a knife around the inside edge of the pan and release the sides. Invert the cake onto a serving plate. Carefully remove the bottom of the cake pan and the parchment paper.

6. Serve the cake sprinkled with some cinnamon and drizzled with a little honey.

CARROT CAKE

Different from your usual carrot cake, this version is made with olive oil and is a bit more savory than most. Serve drizzled with a bit of Greek honey or yogurt for an extra treat.

SERVES 16

⅔ cup olive oil, plus more for greasing
⅓ cup packed light brown sugar
1 pound carrots, grated
2 cups all-purpose flour
1 teaspoon baking soda
1 teaspoon baking powder
1½ teaspoons ground cinnamon
1½ teaspoons ground cloves
1½ cups ground walnuts
½ cup raisins
1 teaspoon vanilla extract
5 eggs

1. Preheat the oven to 350°F. Grease a 9-inch springform pan or an 8 x 10-inch baking pan with a little olive oil.

2. In a large bowl, with an electric mixer, beat the olive oil and brown sugar on high speed until creamy and yellowish in color, 3 to 4 minutes.

3. Stir in the carrots and mix until they are well distributed. Add the flour gradually, beating well after each addition. Add the baking soda, baking powder, cinnamon, cloves, walnuts, raisins, and vanilla. Continue to beat on medium speed until the batter is smooth, 4 to 5 minutes.

4. Add the eggs, one at a time, and beat very well after each addition.

5. Pour the batter into the pan. Bake for 45 to 50 minutes, or until a toothpick inserted into the center of the cake comes out clean.

6. Remove the cake from the oven, allow the cake to cool in the pan, remove from the pan, and serve.

SEMOLINA CAKE (HALVAS)

This cake is among my favorites, because you can control how sweet it is by how much syrup you use. You can also control the flavor profile of the cake this way—try using different juices and spices for variety.

SERVES 16

FOR THE SYRUP
1 cup sugar
Grated zest of 1 orange
2 cups fresh orange juice (about 6 oranges)
1 teaspoon ground cinnamon
A pinch of ground cloves

FOR THE CAKE
1 cup olive oil
1 cup coarse semolina
1 cup fine semolina

½ cup whole blanched almonds

½ cup roasted pine nuts

FOR THE GARNISH

Whole cloves

Blanched whole almonds

Pine nuts

1. Make the syrup: In a saucepan, combine the sugar, orange zest, orange juice, cinnamon, cloves, and 2 cups water. Bring the mixture to a boil, reduce to a simmer, and cook until the sugar dissolves and the syrup is viscous, 6 to 7 minutes. Remove the pot from the heat and use a strainer to remove the orange zest from the syrup. Set aside.

2. Make the cake: In a saucepan, heat the olive oil over medium heat until it is very hot. Using a wooden spoon, stir in both the coarse and fine semolina. Sauté until evenly browned, 4 to 5 minutes. While stirring, carefully ladle the syrup into the semolina. Continue to cook and stir until the syrup is absorbed and the mixture pulls away from the sides of the saucepan. Add the almonds and pine nuts and stir to combine.

3. Transfer the mixture to a nonstick standard-size Bundt cake pan. Allow it to cool for 15 to 20 minutes.

4. Cover the pan with a cake platter, invert the pan, and turn the cake out onto the platter. Garnish the *halvas* with cloves, blanched almonds, and pine nuts.

SNACKS, SAUCES, AND DIPS

MY MOTHER'S GREEK YOGURT

I believe olive oil and yogurt run through my veins. A food staple for my family since childhood, there is no better yogurt recipe than that of my mother. Eaten on its own, used as an ingredient, marinade, or as a garnish, Greek yogurt is the most versatile of all the foods in the Greek Diet's pantry, and my personal favorite.

MAKES APPROXIMATELY 1½ QUARTS

2 quarts plus ¼ cup organic 2% milk
5 tablespoons plain yogurt

1. Remove the milk and the yogurt from the refrigerator and set them aside until they reach room temperature.

2. In a large saucepan, heat 2 quarts of the milk over medium-low heat until it comes to a boil. Pour the boiling milk into a large glass or nonmetal bowl and allow it to cool until it is lukewarm (100° to 105°F) or until a skin forms on the surface of the milk.

3. In a small bowl, combine the yogurt and the remaining ¼ cup milk. Carefully pour the mixture down the sides of the bowl holding the 2 quarts of lukewarm milk, taking care to keep the surface skin of the milk intact by not stirring or jiggling it. Cover the bowl with a clean kitchen towel and set it aside in a warm, dry place overnight (or 8 to 12 hours), until the mixture thickens.

4. Line a fine-mesh sieve with cheesecloth. Holding the sieve over the sink, pour the yogurt into it to drain off any excess liquid. You now have edible yogurt!

5. To transform your homemade yogurt into a thick, creamy Greek yogurt, line a large bowl with cheesecloth (or a clean kitchen towel), allowing the corners of the cloth or towel to hang over the sides of the bowl. Pour the yogurt into the center of the cloth.

6. Twist the four corners of the cloth together to form a bundle of yogurt. Squeeze the bundle as hard as possible over a sink or basin, applying pressure and wringing until there is only a slow drip from the bottom.

7. Using kitchen twine, tie the bundle at the top and place it in a sieve or colander. Put the sieve with the bundle back in the bowl, taking care that the bundle does not touch the bottom of the bowl. Refrigerate the bowl holding the yogurt bundle for 2 to 3 hours.

8. Remove the bundle from the refrigerator and squeeze it again over the sink, applying as much pressure as possible with the palms of your hands to remove any remaining liquid. When you're confident you've squeezed out as much liquid as possible, untie the bundle. Using a spoon or spatula, spoon the yogurt into a bowl or glass container. Store in the refrigerator until ready to eat.

Cook's note: The yogurt will keep for 4 to 5 days in the refrigerator. Be sure to save a little before it's all gone so you can make your next batch of homemade yogurt!

MARIA'S HUMMUS

Hummus has become one of the most important foods of the modern day. Packed full of protein, vitamins, and flavor, it's great for snacking on any time, or using as a condiment for just about anything! Feel free to make your own flavor combination by adding different herbs and spices or vegetables!

MAKES 2½ TO 3 CUPS

1 red bell pepper
2 cups dried chickpeas or one 16-ounce can chickpeas
1 teaspoon baking soda (if using dried chickpeas)
1 medium onion, quartered
2 garlic cloves, peeled
¼ cup tahini
2 to 3 tablespoons fresh lemon juice
Red pepper flakes (optional)
½ cup extra-virgin olive oil, plus more for drizzling
Salt
Warmed whole-grain pita bread and/or crudités, for serving

1. Roast the pepper by placing it over an open flame at medium-high heat on your stovetop. Rotate it consistently using tongs until the entire outside is charred, about 10 to 15 minutes. Place in a bowl, cover with plastic wrap, and allow to steam for 15 minutes. Remove the pepper from the bowl, peel the skin using your hands, remove the seed, and chop. Set aside.

2. If you're using canned chickpeas, skip to Step 4. If you are using dried chickpeas, place them in a medium pot. Cover the chickpeas with water, stir in the baking soda, and allow them to soak overnight.

3. The next day, rinse and drain the soaked dried chickpeas. Heat a medium pot over medium heat until hot. Add the chickpeas, onion, and enough water to cover the contents of the pot by 3 inches. Cover the pot and bring to a boil. Reduce the heat to a simmer and continue to cook the chickpeas for about 45 minutes, skimming as needed to remove foam, until soft. Drain the chickpeas and reserve the onion. Allow the chickpeas to cool.

4. If using canned chickpeas, sauté the onion over medium heat until translucent, about 5 minutes. Combine the roasted red pepper, garlic, and tahini in a food processor or blender. Process, scraping down the sides of

the processor as necessary, until smooth. Add the chickpeas, sautéed onion (or reserved onion if using soaked chickpeas), lemon juice, and pepper flakes (if using). Process, scraping down the sides again if necessary, until smooth. With the machine running, gradually add the ½ cup olive oil and process until the mixture is emulsified. Add salt to taste and more pepper flakes, if desired. Spoon the hummus into a serving dish.

5. To serve, drizzle with extra-virgin olive oil and pair with warm whole-grain pita bread and/or fresh crudités, including celery, carrots, and sliced red and green peppers.

TZATZIKI

Tzatziki is one of the most well-known Greek condiments available, and for good reason—it pairs perfectly with most foods, and adds a healthy, herbaceous kick to anything it touches. You'll see it referenced throughout these recipes, so don't hesitate to get a little experimental and have some fun! We recommend serving the tzatziki as a sauce for vegetables, chicken, pasta, or eggs, or as an appetizer with crudités or grilled whole-grain pita.

MAKES 2 TO 3 CUPS

2 cucumbers
Salt
16 ounces 2% plain Greek yogurt
3 garlic cloves, peeled
3 tablespoons extra-virgin olive oil
2 tablespoons red wine vinegar
3 to 4 sprigs of fresh dill, stems removed and roughly chopped, or 1 teaspoon dried dill

1. Peel the cucumbers. Using the large holes of a box grater, grate them into a sieve or colander. Lightly salt the grated cucumber (this helps draw out the moisture), cover the sieve with plastic wrap, and allow the cucumber to drain overnight. (Note: Placing a heavy plate or glass on top of the covered cucumbers will help the draining process.)

2. In a large bowl, combine the drained cucumber and yogurt. Mix very well. Using a Microplane grater or a small, sharp knife, grate or mince the garlic. Stir the garlic into the yogurt mixture. Stir in the olive oil and vinegar and mix well. Cover the bowl with plastic and refrigerate for about 1 hour.

3. Stir in the dill and refrigerate until serving.

EGGPLANT SALAD (MELITZANOSALATA)

One of the things I love about eggplant is the luscious mouthfeel is gives any dish that uses it. My eggplant salad is the essence of what that feeling is all about, seemingly rich and fatty, but actually nutritious and delicious. Add some extra herbs and spices, or some feta or Greek yogurt to elevate this recipe even more! Serve with warm whole-grain pita bread or as a dip for crudités.

MAKES 4 TO 5 CUPS

3 pounds eggplants
½ cup extra-virgin olive oil
3 tablespoons fresh lemon juice
2 garlic cloves, minced
Salt
Sprigs of fresh parsley, for garnish

1. Preheat a grill or a grill pan over medium-high heat until very hot. Place the eggplants on the grill or grill pan and grill, rotating often, until they are evenly softened and charred, 10 to 15 minutes. (Alternatively, you can roast the whole eggplants by placing them on a baking sheet lined with parchment paper and baking them in a preheated 375°F oven for 15 to 20 minutes, or until softened.)

2. Transfer the grilled or roasted eggplants to a large glass bowl and cover the bowl with plastic wrap, or place the eggplants in a zip-seal plastic bag. Let them steam for 10 minutes.

3. Peel the eggplants and halve them lengthwise to remove the seeds (optional). Cut the eggplants into small chunks 1 to 2 inches in diameter (the size isn't important as you'll be mashing them later). Place the eggplant chunks into a sieve and set the sieve aside over a large plate to drain for 10 to 15 minutes.

4. Transfer the eggplant chunks back to the large bowl. Mash them lightly, using two forks, until they resemble a coarse puree. Slowly alternate pouring in the olive oil and the lemon juice, stirring constantly, until well blended.

5. Stir in the garlic, and season to taste with salt. Cover the bowl with plastic wrap and refrigerate for at least 2 hours.

6. Stir the eggplant salad thoroughly, garnish it with parsley sprigs, and serve.

WALNUT-OLIVE SPREAD

Walnuts are earthy, rich nuts with a great deal of character. Olives are the fruit of Greece, briny and bright. In this recipe, they come together with some supporting herbs and spices to create a well-balanced spread ideal for topping off pastas, eggs, chicken, fish, and meat. Try it with Grilled Chicken Breast (Kotopoulo Psito) (page 246).

MAKES 3 TO 4 CUPS

2 cups pitted, finely chopped kalamata olives
2 cups finely chopped, toasted walnuts (see Cook's note)
½ cup finely chopped red bell pepper
2 tablespoons dried oregano
¼ cup stemmed, chopped fresh mint
2 teaspoons red pepper flakes
About ¼ cup extra-virgin olive oil
Salt and freshly ground black pepper
Whole-Grain Pita Chips (page 281) or rustic bread, for serving

1. Combine the olives, walnuts, bell pepper, oregano, mint, and pepper flakes in a food processor or a blender. Slowly drizzle in enough olive oil just to cover. Process the mixture until smooth. It should be the consistency of natural chunky peanut butter. Add a little more olive oil if necessary. Season to taste with salt and pepper.

2. Transfer the spread to a serving bowl and allow it to sit for at least 10 minutes. The longer it rests, the better it tastes. It can sit out for about 30 minutes before serving.

3. Refrigerate the spread if not serving immediately, and bring it to room temperature before serving. Serve the spread with pita chips or slices of rustic bread.

Cook's note: To toast walnuts, preheat the oven to 375°F. Line a baking sheet with foil or parchment paper. Spread the walnuts on the baking sheet and roast for 5 to 10 minutes, stirring often, or until they start to brown and develop a nutty aroma.

TARAMOSALATA (CARP ROE SPREAD)

Taramosalata is one of my favorite recipes to make, because it's easy, and because it's science in action. Taking a liquid and turning it into a solid with the help of a few binding agents exemplifies the magic of a true emulsion. The flavors are bright and tangy, reminiscent of the sea, and the creamy texture is indulgent in and of itself. Truly Greek in nature, this famous spread has it all.

MAKES 2½ TO 3 CUPS

1 cup white tarama (see Cook's note)
¼ small white or red onion (or use a shallot instead)
2 cups extra-virgin olive oil
2 tablespoons fresh lemon juice
Lemon rounds, for garnish
Kalamata olives, for garnish
Whole-Grain Pita Bread (page 280), Whole-Grain Pita Chips (page 281), or romaine lettuce, for serving

1. Desalt the *tarama* by placing the roe in a bowl of water to cover and setting it aside for 1 hour. Drain the roe and set aside.

2. Puree the onion in a food processor or a blender. Add the tarama and blend until the mixture is creamy. With the machine running, gradually add the olive oil. Gradually add the lemon juice and continue to blend until the mixture is thick and smooth. Taste the taramosalata, and season it to taste with additional lemon juice or pureed onion.

3. Transfer the taramosalata to a bowl and garnish it with lemon rounds and olives. Serve it with pita bread or pita chips, or on a bed of romaine lettuce.

Cook's note: Tarama is carp roe. If you can't find it at the market, talk to your local fishmonger, or order it online.

ROASTED BEET–YOGURT DIP

This colorful dip is full of flavor and personality, hitting all the different notes on your palate! The roasted beets add the sweetness, the jalapeño has the heat, the lemon juice brightens it with acid, and the combination of ingredients gives us the saltiness we crave. Eat this with homemade Whole-Grain Pita Chips (page 281) or Zucchini Croquettes (page 211).

MAKES ABOUT 4 CUPS

2 pounds beets
Olive oil, for coating the beets
Salt and freshly ground black pepper
1 cup 2% plain Greek yogurt
2 cloves garlic, grated
5 tablespoons Greek olive oil
2 tablespoons fresh lemon juice
1 small red onion, finely chopped
1 jalapeño chile pepper, seeded and finely chopped
Leaves from 3 sprigs of fresh mint, chopped

1. The night before you plan to serve this dip, preheat the oven to 400°F. Scrub the beets thoroughly and place them in a large bowl. Toss with enough olive oil to coat them, and sprinkle them with some salt and pepper.

2. Transfer the beets to a small roasting pan, cover the pan with foil, and roast for 1½ to 2 hours, or until the beets are very soft. To test for doneness, poke the beets with the tines of a fork.

3. Allow the beets to cool thoroughly. Peel the beets, roughly chop them, and transfer to a medium bowl. Cover the bowl and refrigerate it overnight.

4. The next day, in a large bowl, stir together the yogurt, garlic, olive oil, and lemon juice. Mix well with a large spoon until all the ingredients are well combined.

5. In a large blender or food processor, puree the beets until very smooth. Fold the pureed beets into the yogurt mixture. Stir in the red onion and jalapeño, mixing thoroughly.

6. Cover the bowl of dip with plastic wrap and refrigerate it for at least 1 hour. Just before serving, sprinkle the dip with the mint, stirring until the mint is well incorporated.

MINT-YOGURT SAUCE

Bright and refreshing, this sauce pairs with almost anything! Try it with freshly grilled souvlaki (pages 192, 239, 245, and 254), grilled chicken or fish, or with a fresh piece of Multigrain Bread (page 282)!

MAKES ABOUT 2 CUPS

2 cups 2% plain Greek yogurt

¼ cup chopped fresh mint leaves (no stems)

2 tablespoons fresh lemon juice

2 teaspoons Greek olive oil

Salt and freshly ground black pepper

1. In a large bowl, combine the yogurt, mint, lemon juice, and olive oil. Whisk thoroughly.

2. Season to taste with salt and pepper before serving.

TRADITIONAL EGG-LEMON SAUCE (AVGOLEMONO SAUCE)

Avgolemono sauce is not as scary or complicated a sauce as people think it is; the key to making my special recipe has to do with tempering the eggs, so it will not curdle when added to another dish!

MAKES ABOUT 2 CUPS

2 eggs

2 tablespoons gluten-free flour or all-purpose flour

2 cups cold water

Juice of 1 lemon (2 to 3 tablespoons)

1. In a saucepan, vigorously whisk the eggs and flour until fully combined. Continuing to whisk, add the cold water slowly.

2. Place the saucepan over low heat and, while still whisking, slowly add the lemon juice. Continue to cook over low heat, whisking constantly, until the mixture becomes creamy. When it has a thick, silky texture, remove the sauce from the heat.

3. Add this sauce to recipes that call for it, and use it to finish any dish that you want to have a luscious, lemony kick!

LADOLEMONO SAUCE

Ladolemono is the most ubiquitous sauce in the Greek culinary arsenal. Used for everything from salad dressing to a finishing sauce, from integral to optional, this simple sauce pairs perfectly with pretty much everything!

MAKES ABOUT 1½ CUPS

⅓ cup fresh lemon juice (2 to 3 lemons)
¼ teaspoon mustard powder
Salt and freshly ground black pepper
1 cup extra-virgin olive oil

1. In a tightly resealable container, combine the lemon juice, mustard powder, and salt and pepper to taste. Cover and shake vigorously until fully combined.

2. Add the olive oil, cover the container, and shake vigorously until the sauce has emulsified.

CARAMELIZED TOMATOES (AND COULIS)

These caramelized tomatoes serve as the base for many of my recipes—sweet and slightly acidic with great roasted flavor, they lend perfect balance to anything that incorporates them.

MAKES ABOUT 2 CUPS COULIS

10 plum tomatoes
1 tablespoon dried oregano
2 tablespoons light brown sugar
Salt and freshly ground black pepper
1 bunch seedless green grapes (approximately 1 cup), finely chopped
½ cup balsamic vinegar
⅓ cup olive oil

1. Preheat the oven to 350°F. Line a large baking sheet with parchment paper.

2. Quarter the tomatoes lengthwise, remove the seeds, and arrange them, skin side down, on the baking sheet. Sprinkle them with the oregano and brown sugar. Season liberally with salt and pepper. Top the tomatoes with the finely chopped grapes and sprinkle first with the balsamic vinegar and then with the olive oil.

3. Roast the tomatoes for about 40 minutes, or until they darken in color and the edges look roasted.

4. If making the coulis, transfer the roasted tomatoes (grapes and all) to a food processor or high-speed blender and blend until smooth.

BAKED KALE CHIPS

The ancient Greeks were known to eat kale to help ease a hangover, but in modern times, we eat it because it's a delicious, cruciferous superfood! These baked kale chips are great for snacking and highly addictive—use your favorite spices to make your own unique flavor!

SERVES 6

1 bunch curly kale
1 or 2 tablespoons olive oil
Salt
Optional seasonings: garlic powder, cayenne pepper, dried oregano, sumac, or other ground spices

1. Preheat the oven to 350°F. Line a large baking sheet with parchment paper.

2. Using your hands or a pair of kitchen shears, carefully remove the thick stems from the kale. Tear or cut the leaves into bite-size pieces.

3. Using a salad spinner, thoroughly wash and dry the kale pieces. Transfer the kale to a large bowl, drizzle it with olive oil, and sprinkle it with salt and whatever optional seasonings you like.

4. Transfer the kale to the baking sheet and bake for 10 to 15 minutes, or until the edges are browned but not burned. If you don't eat all the kale chips right away, store them in an airtight container.

BAKED APPLE CHIPS

One of my favorite ways to eat apples, these chips are a wonderful snacking alternative to fit the old adage "an apple a day keeps the doctor away." If you like, substitute pears for apples and enjoy homemade pear chips!

SERVES 2

2 crisp apples, such as Granny Smith, Pink Lady, or Braeburn
Cinnamon, as needed

1. Preheat the oven to 275°F. Line a large baking sheet with parchment paper.

2. Core and slice the apples as thinly as possible. It's not necessary to peel them. The easiest way to get paper-thin slices is to use a mandoline.

3. Arrange the apple slices on the baking sheet, sprinkle lightly with cinnamon, and bake them for about 1 hour. Using a large spatula or spoon, flip the slices over and continue to bake for another hour, stirring them again after 30 minutes, until they are crisp.

4. Remove the apple chips from the oven and allow them to cool on the baking sheet for another 15 to 20 minutes to develop more crispiness.

CRUNCHY TOASTED CHICKPEAS

These crunchy chickpeas are great to take with you on the go, and are versatile enough to be eaten as is, or used as a garnish for a dish that needs some texture. You can add any spices you like to create your own original flavor combinations!

SERVES 4

One 16-ounce can chickpeas, rinsed and drained
2 tablespoons olive oil
Salt
Optional seasonings: garlic powder, cayenne pepper, ground cumin

1. Preheat the oven to 425°F. Line a baking sheet with parchment paper.

2. Blot the chickpeas with a paper towel to remove as much moisture as possible.

3. In a bowl, toss the chickpeas with the olive oil. Season with salt to taste. If you like, season with garlic powder, cayenne pepper, and ground cumin, or any other spices you enjoy, and toss to ensure even dispersion.

4. Spread the seasoned chickpeas out on the baking sheet. Bake for 30 to 40 minutes, or until browned and crunchy. Be sure to keep an eye on them for the last 10 minutes, to avoid burning. Remove from the oven and allow them to cool and crisp up before serving.

WHOLE-GRAIN PITA BREAD

The ultimate in Greek culinary necessities, pita bread can be found accompanying nearly every meal. Use this recipe to complement souvlaki (pages 192, 239, 245, and 254) or as a vehicle for consuming delicious dips like Tzatziki (page 271), Taramosalata (page 274), and Maria's Hummus (page 270).

SERVES 12

1½ cups warm water
2 tablespoons olive oil
1½ teaspoons active dry yeast (from 1 packet)
1 teaspoon salt
1 teaspoon sugar
1½ cups all-purpose flour
2 cups whole wheat flour
Cornmeal, for dusting
Olive oil, for coating the pan

1. In a large bowl, combine the water, olive oil, yeast, salt, and sugar. Stir to combine. Allow to stand for 5 minutes or until the yeast bubbles slightly, a sign that it is active.

2. Using your hands, gradually add the flours to the bowl. Knead the mixture with your hands until it forms a dough that pulls cleanly away from the sides of the bowl. Cover the bowl and set it aside in a warm spot in the kitchen for about 2 hours.

3. Preheat the oven to 350°F.

4. Divide the dough into 12 equal portions. Roll out each portion into a 6- to 8-inch round. Each pita should be about ¼ inch thick. Dust both sides of each pita lightly with cornmeal. Poke the surface of each pita with the tines of a fork, taking care not to poke all the way through the dough.

5. Rub a large, heavy cast-iron skillet or baking pan with olive oil. Place it in the hot oven to preheat for 7 to 10 minutes.

6. Arrange some of the pita in the hot skillet in a single layer. Bake them in batches for about 15 minutes, or until they puff up.

7. Serve the pita bread warm, or allow them to cool on a large tray lined with a kitchen towel. Transfer them to a plastic bag, seal the bag, and use within 1 week. Or you may freeze the pita bread, in the sealed plastic bag, for up to 3 months.

WHOLE-GRAIN PITA CHIPS

These multipurpose whole-grain pita chips are a quick and easy way to make pita that is past its prime useful again! Feel free to add different herbs and/or spices to make your own version of flavored pita chips. (My favorite is garlic and thyme!)

Whole-Grain Pita Bread (page 280)
Olive oil, for brushing
Salt and freshly ground black pepper

1. Preheat the oven to 400°F.

2. Cut the pita bread into whatever size chips you'd like and arrange them on a baking sheet (lined with parchment paper, if desired).

3. Brush the chips lightly with olive oil, season them lightly with salt and pepper, and bake for 5 to 8 minutes, or until they are crispy.

MULTIGRAIN BREAD (OF THE ANCIENT GREEKS)

This recipe can be found in my book *Ancient Dining,* the official cookbook for the Athens 2004 Olympic Games (ISP International Athletic Editions, 2004). The ancient Greeks would make this bread to eat with nearly every meal, whether accompanied by olive oil, beans, or fruit.

SERVES 10 TO 12

1 ounce fresh yeast (equivalent to 1 cake)

1 cup lukewarm water

1 cup 2% plain Greek yogurt

1 tablespoon honey

½ teaspoon salt

5 cups whole wheat flour

1 cup all-purpose flour

3 tablespoons olive oil, plus more for kneading and baking

1 tablespoon plus 1 teaspoon poppyseeds

1 tablespoon plus 1 teaspoon 1 flax seeds

1 tablespoon plus 1 teaspoon sesame seeds

1 tablespoon plus 1 teaspoon pumpkin or sunflower seeds

1. In a large bowl, dissolve the yeast in the lukewarm water. Add the yogurt, honey, and salt and stir to thoroughly combine.

2. Gradually add the flours, along with 3 tablespoons olive oil and 1 tablespoon *each* of the poppyseeds, flax seeds, sesame seeds, and pumpkin or sunflower seeds.

3. Begin to knead the dough by hand, occasionally dipping your fingers into a little olive oil to keep the dough from sticking. Continue kneading for 10 minutes, or until the dough becomes fluffy and smooth.

4. Transfer the dough to a large greased bowl and set it aside in a warm place for 30 minutes to 1 hour to rest and rise until approximately doubled in size.

5. Repeat the kneading process, then shape the dough into 1 or 2 loaves or into buns. This is a free-form recipe, so the rolls can be any size you like, and shaped round to braided. Sprinkle the top with the remaining seeds.

6. Place the loaves or rolls on a lightly oiled baking pan large enough to hold them in a single layer and to allow for some expansion. Allow the rolls or loaves to proof in a warm place, covered, for about 1 hour. When they have risen, they're ready to bake.

7. Preheat the oven to 350°F.

8. Bake the bread for about 1 hour, or until the crust is golden brown. The rolls will take substantially less time, but the length of baking will depend upon how large they are. The crust should be hard and have a good "knock" to it. Remove the bread or rolls from the oven, and allow to cool for 20 to 30 minutes. Remove from the baking pan.

Cook's note: This recipe may require a little more water or flour, depending on the moisture in the air, the elevation, and the time of year—all these factors affect the absorption potential of flour.

GREEK COFFEE

There are many different ideas on how to make the best cup of Greek coffee, but for me, this is the best!

1. To a briki (a small copper or brass pot specially made to brew Greek coffee), add as much cold water as the number of cups of coffee you want to make.

2. For every 2 ounces of water, add 1 heaping teaspoon of Greek coffee. (If you like your coffee stronger, add more coffee!)

3. Place the briki directly over a low flame, constantly stirring until it boils. When it boils, you'll see brown froth rise to the top of the briki. At this point, remove it from the heat, and gently knock it on a flat surface to allow the grinds to settle to the bottom of the pot. It's ready to serve.

Cook's note: If you like sugar in your coffee (I don't), add your sugar to the coffee before boiling it. If you like milk in your coffee (I don't), add it after you boil it, but make sure the milk is warm!

GREEK MOUNTAIN TEA

Greek mountain tea is incredibly easy to make, because it's all about the method.

SERVES 1 TO 2

1. The tea comes as flowers and stems sealed in a package. Take about one-quarter of the bag, break up the stems and flowers, and add it to a pot.

2. Fill the pot with water and slowly bring the water to a boil, allowing the tea to steep from the beginning. The longer the tea is in the water, the stronger and more flavorful the tea will be!

3. You can serve it strained or with the flowers and stems in the cup, with honey and lemon or milk. (The combination of honey and lemon is great for absorbing the iron in the tea!)

4. My favorite is to brew the tea, allow it to cool, then refrigerate for an hour, and drink it iced all day long!

GREEK MORNING SHAKE

Rich, luscious, and satisfying, this simple shake will start your day off right!

SERVES 4

1 cup ice
2 cups 2% plain Greek yogurt
1 cup brewed Greek Coffee (page 283)
2 tablespoons honey
1 cup 2% milk

1. In a blender, blend the ice until it is crushed.

2. Add the yogurt, coffee, honey, and milk to the crushed ice. Blend until smooth. Pour into glasses.

ACKNOWLEDGMENTS

WE COULD NOT HAVE WRITTEN *The Greek Diet* without the enthusiastic, intelligent, and continual input of Chef Dara Davenport. Dara spent many long days with us poring over pages and mixing up recipes. Her clever suggestions and wit have added immensely to the authenticity and beauty of this book.

We are also indebted to registered dietician Georgia Giannapoulos for her nutritional insight and hard work in helping us create *The Greek Diet* menu plans. Thank you, too, to agent Alan Morell, who helped set this book in motion and remained a solid compass throughout.

There is no better publishing team than the triad at HarperCollins: Lisa Sharkey, Amy Bendell, and Paige Hazzan. Their editorial direction and patience have been the stuff of Greek goddesses—our enduring thanks to you.

To Dr. Nikolaides, thank you for the heartfelt reminder to look back to Greek traditions and my grandmother's recipes. To the Chef's Club of Greece and president Miltos Karoumbas, thank you for naming Maria the official ambassador of Greek gastronomy—you have entrusted the right chef to share Greek cuisine with the world! And Maria's culinary colleagues have helped to guide her down the path to good food and wonderful health: *yiassou* to Elena Reppa, Ioannis Nasopoulos, Konstantinos Vlachos, and Ioannis Tompas, and walking partner Jim Niforos.

And most of all, thank you to Maria's family, who raised her to believe in herself, her heritage, and the healing power of traditional, great-tasting food.

INDEX

About the Authors

MARIA LOI, international ambassador of Greek gastronomy, restaurateur, and public personality, is widely regarded as "the Martha Stewart of Greece." The author of multiple cookbooks, including the official cookbook for the Athens 2004 Olympic Games, Maria is known to be the authority on Greek cuisine. Maria has cooked at the White House for President Barack Obama, Vice President Joe Biden, and 250 guests. She opened Loi Estiatorio in the heart of Manhattan to rave reviews. Maria also takes pride in philanthropic work; she is a founder of Elpida, a foundation to support children with cancer.

SARAH TOLAND is a longtime health and nutrition journalist and former professional track-and-field athlete. She is currently the food and nutrition director of *Prevention* magazine and has appeared regularly as a weight-loss expert for Fox News Channel. Sarah also served as the senior health editor of *Men's Journal* and *Alternative Medicine*, the editor in chief of *Inside Triathlon*, and has written on health and fitness for the *New York Times* and *Sports Illustrated*, among other national publications.